Birds

White-throated Hummingbird

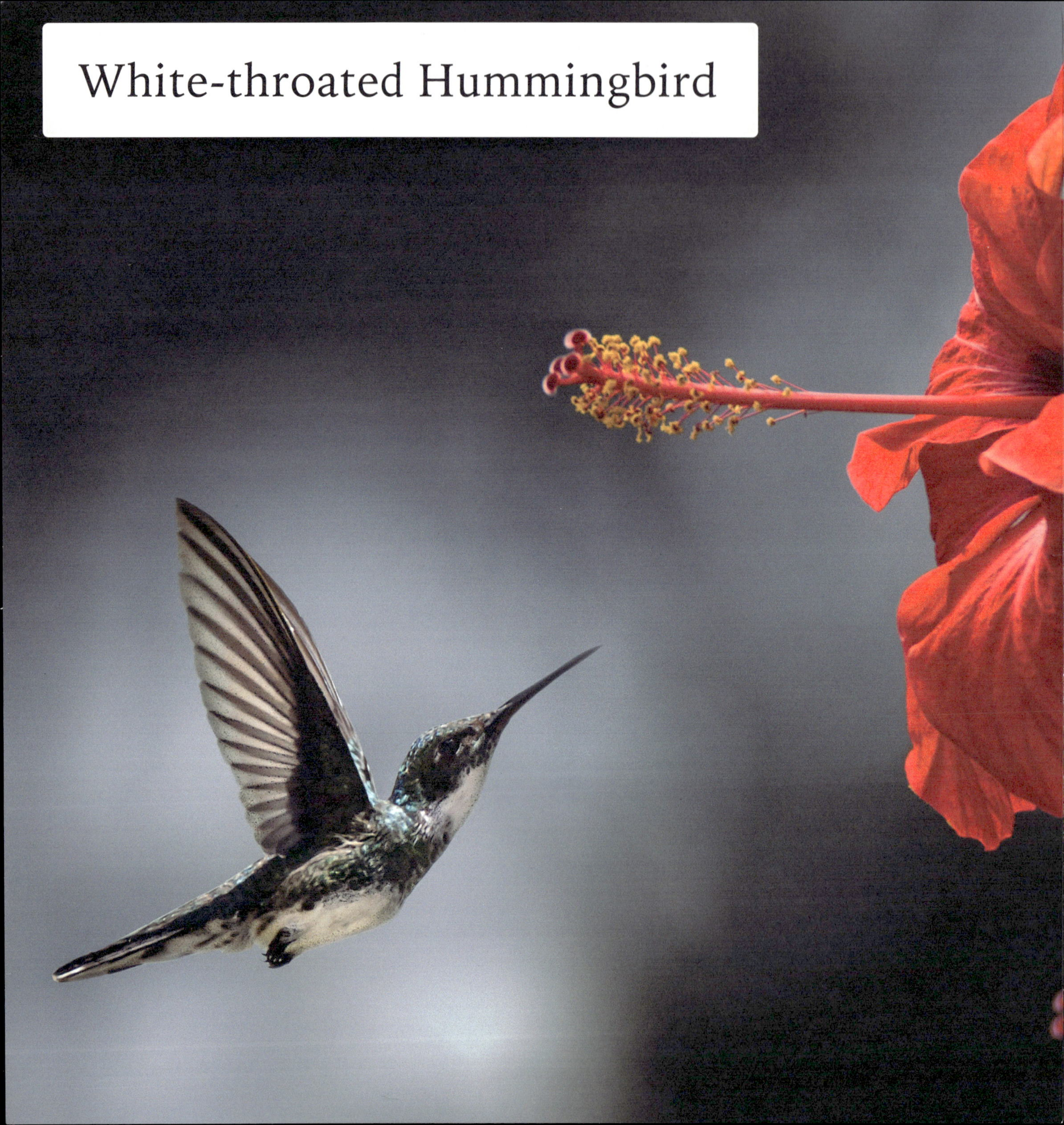

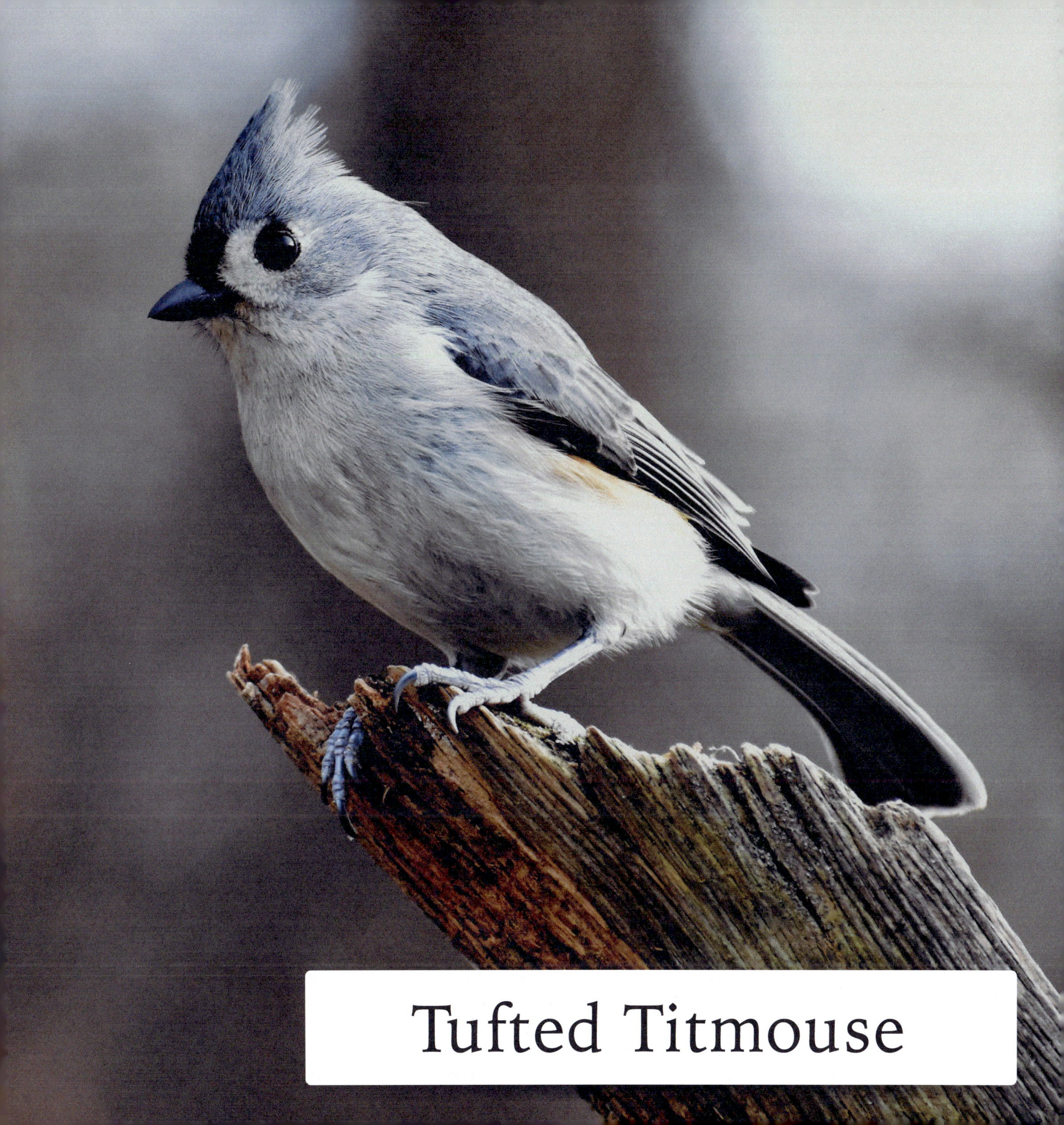

Tufted Titmouse

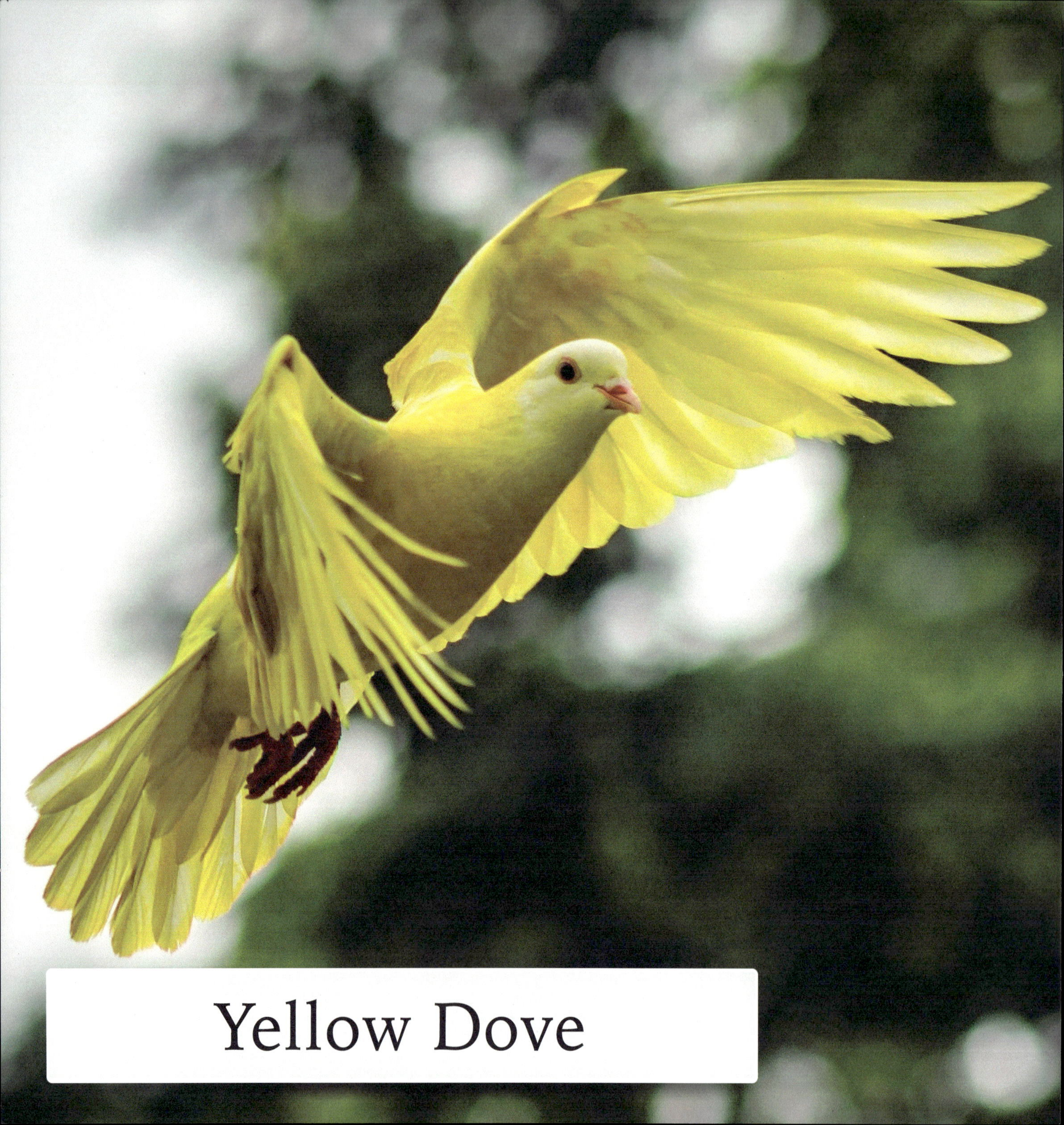

Yellow Dove

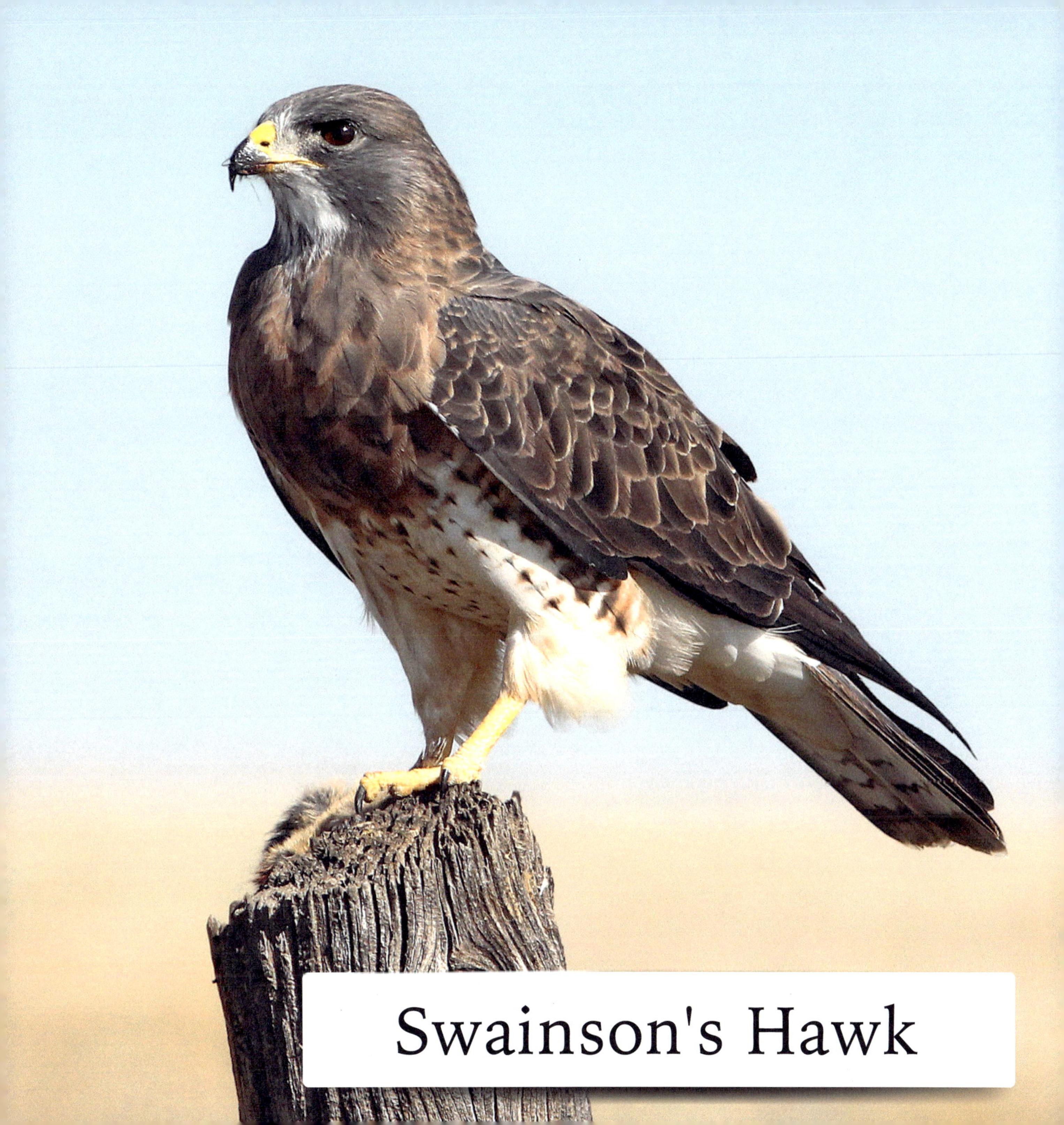

Swainson's Hawk

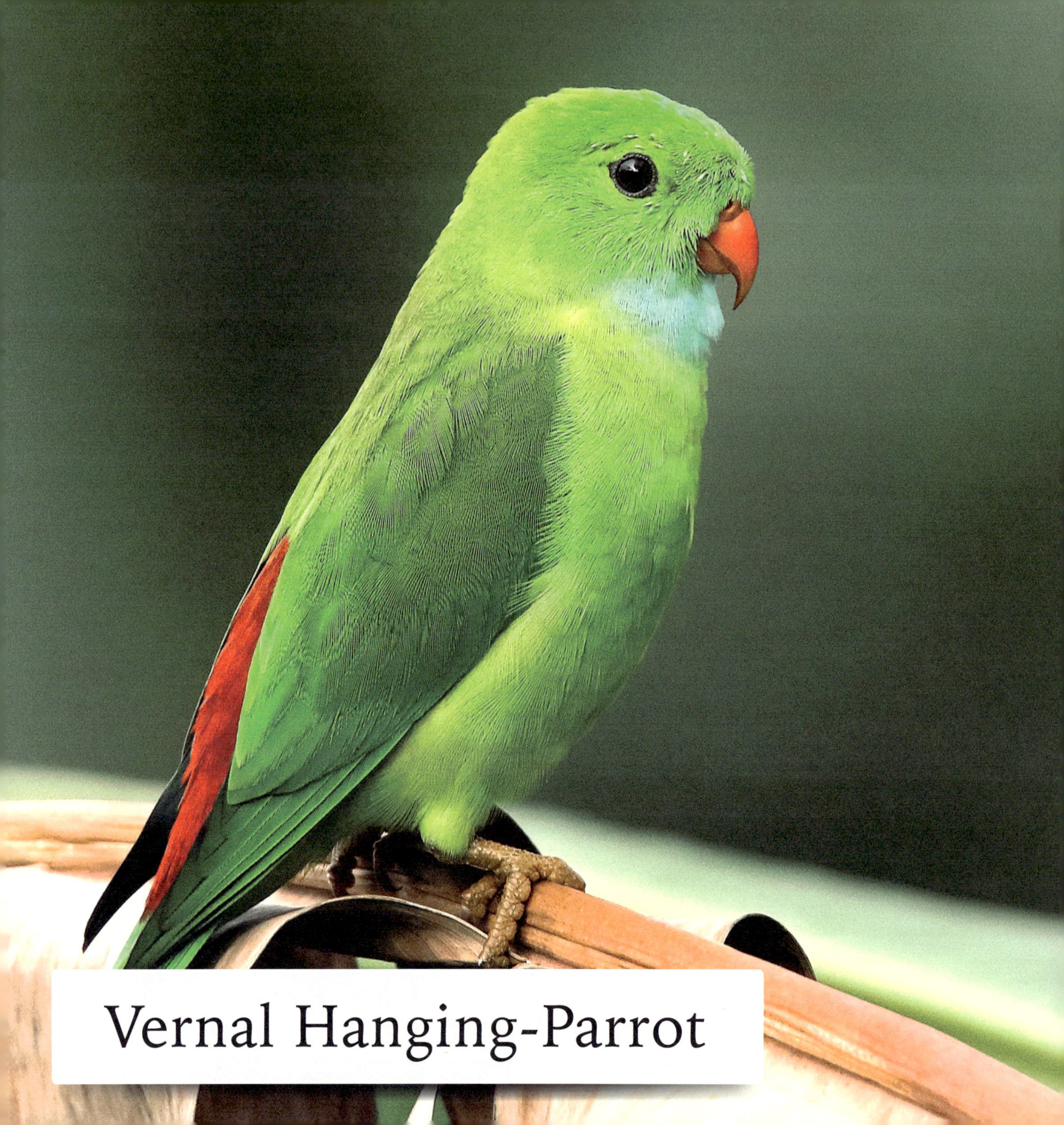

Vernal Hanging-Parrot

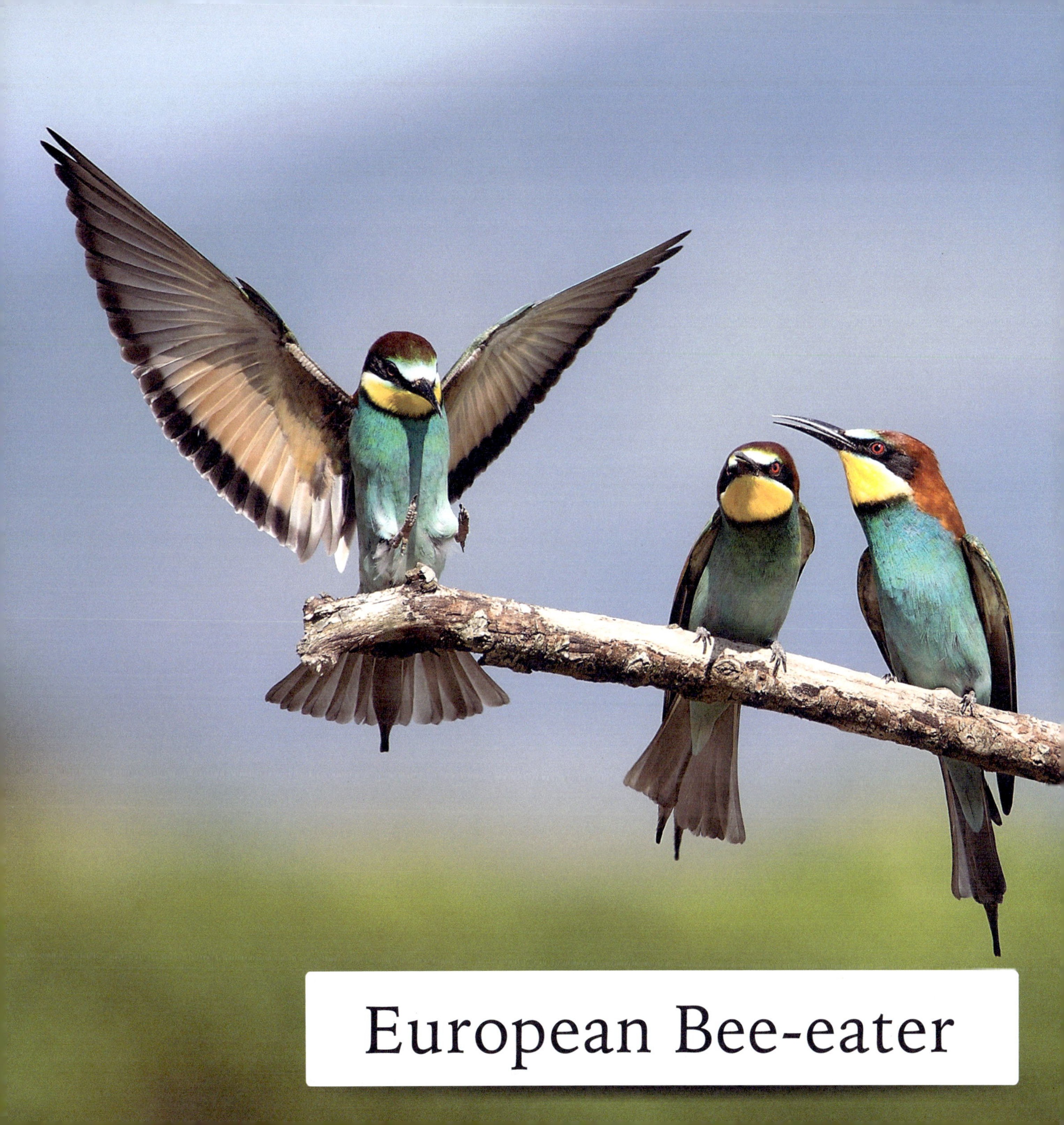

European Bee-eater

Indian Peafowl

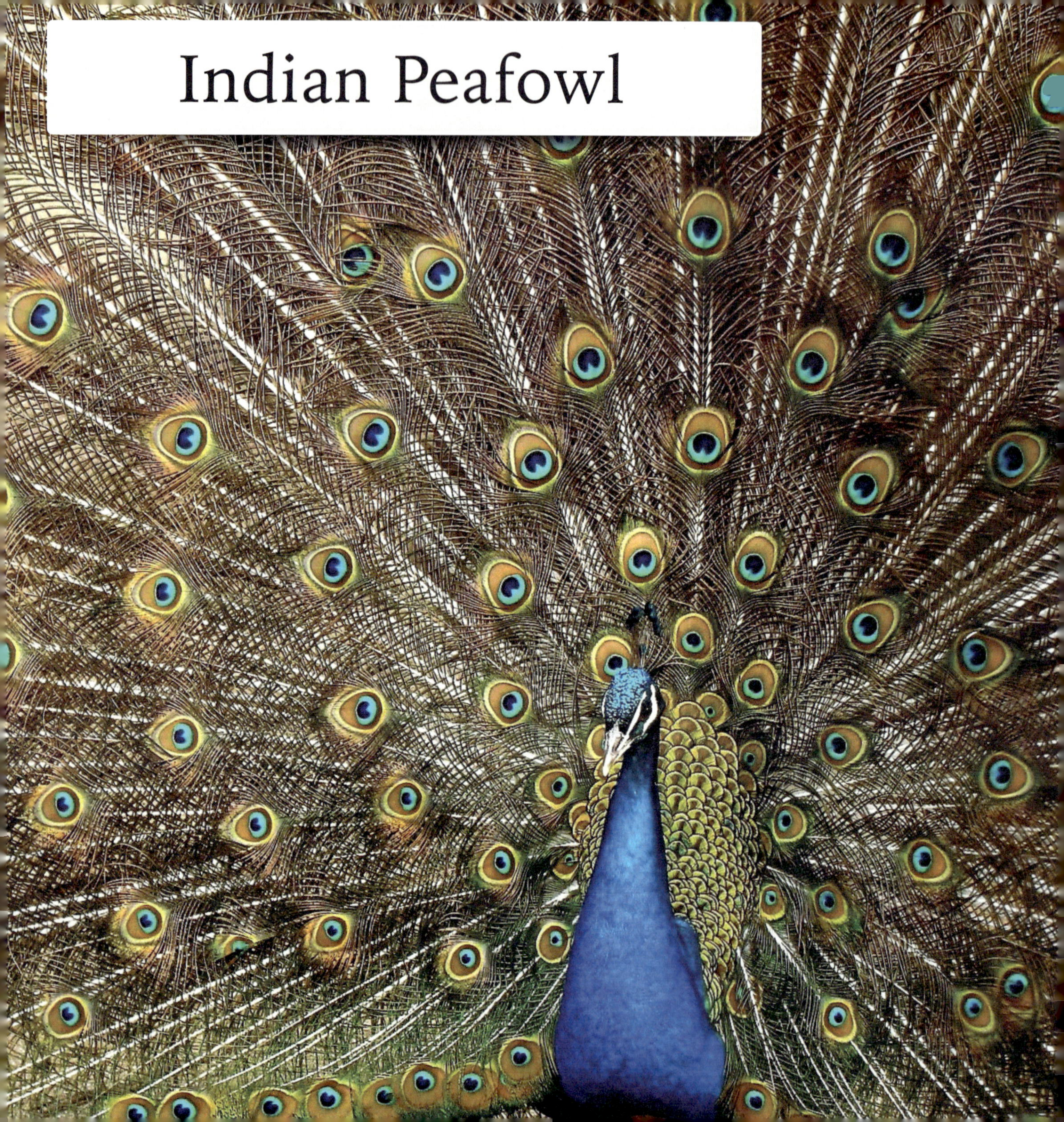

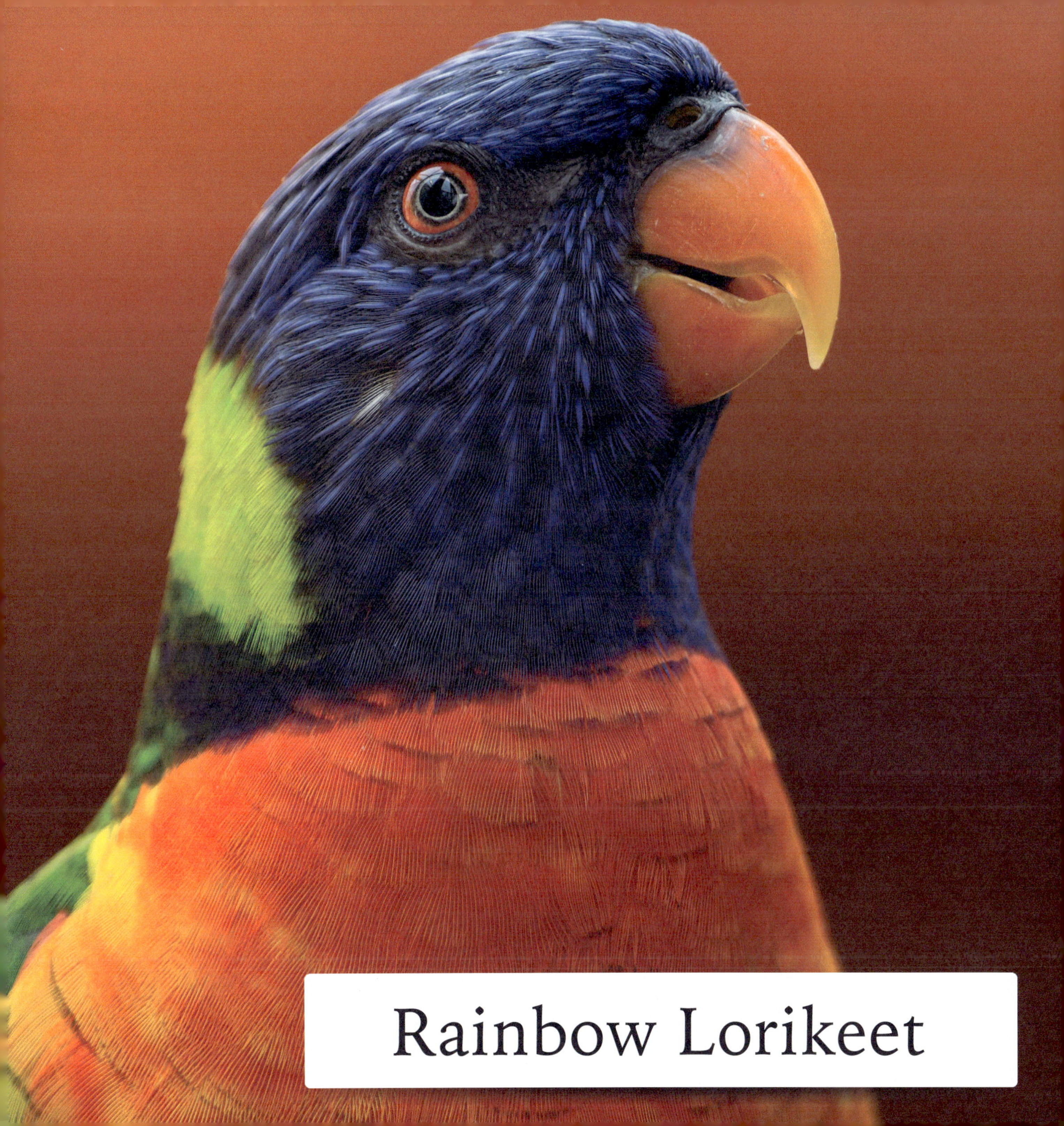

Rainbow Lorikeet

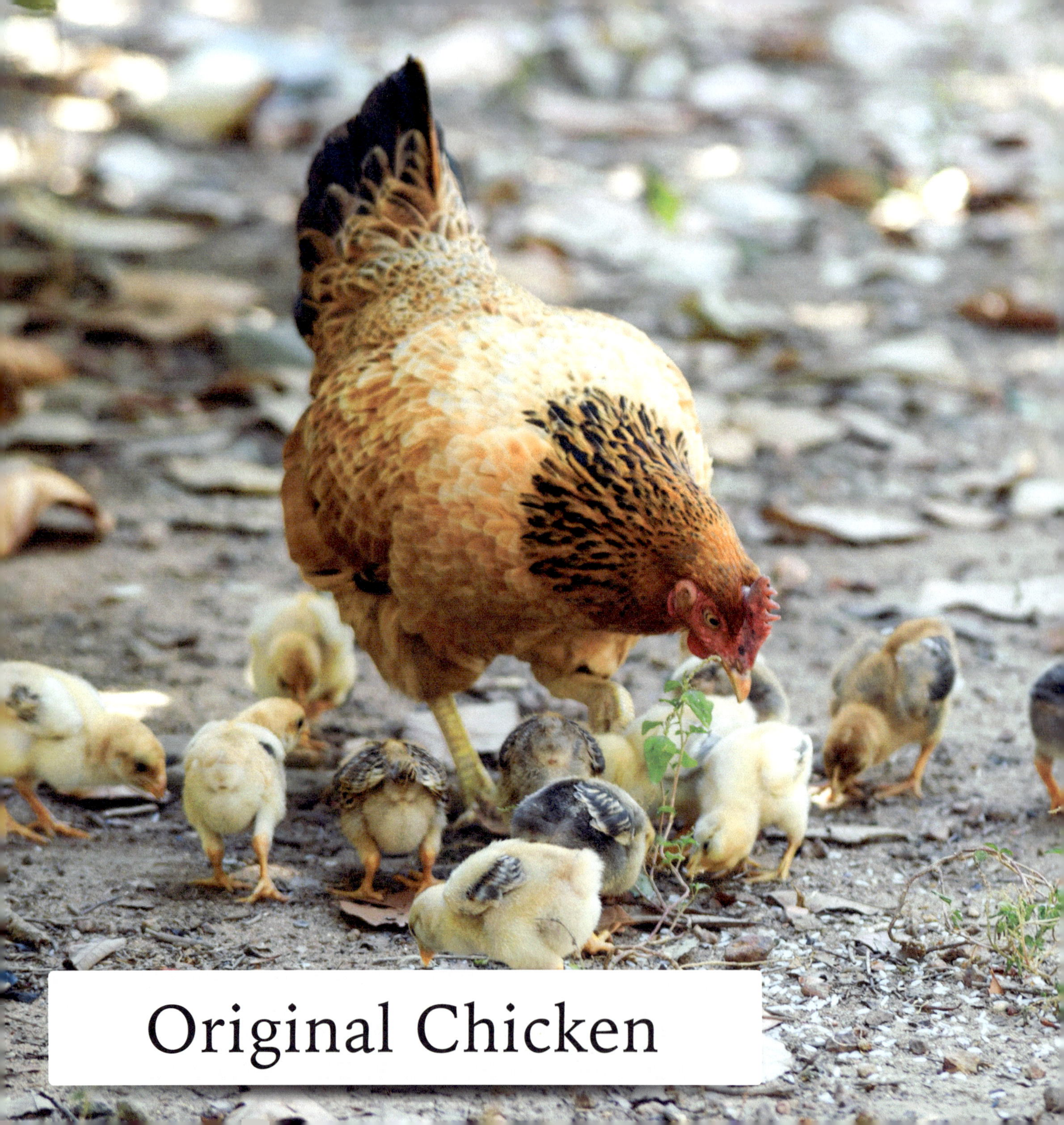

Original Chicken

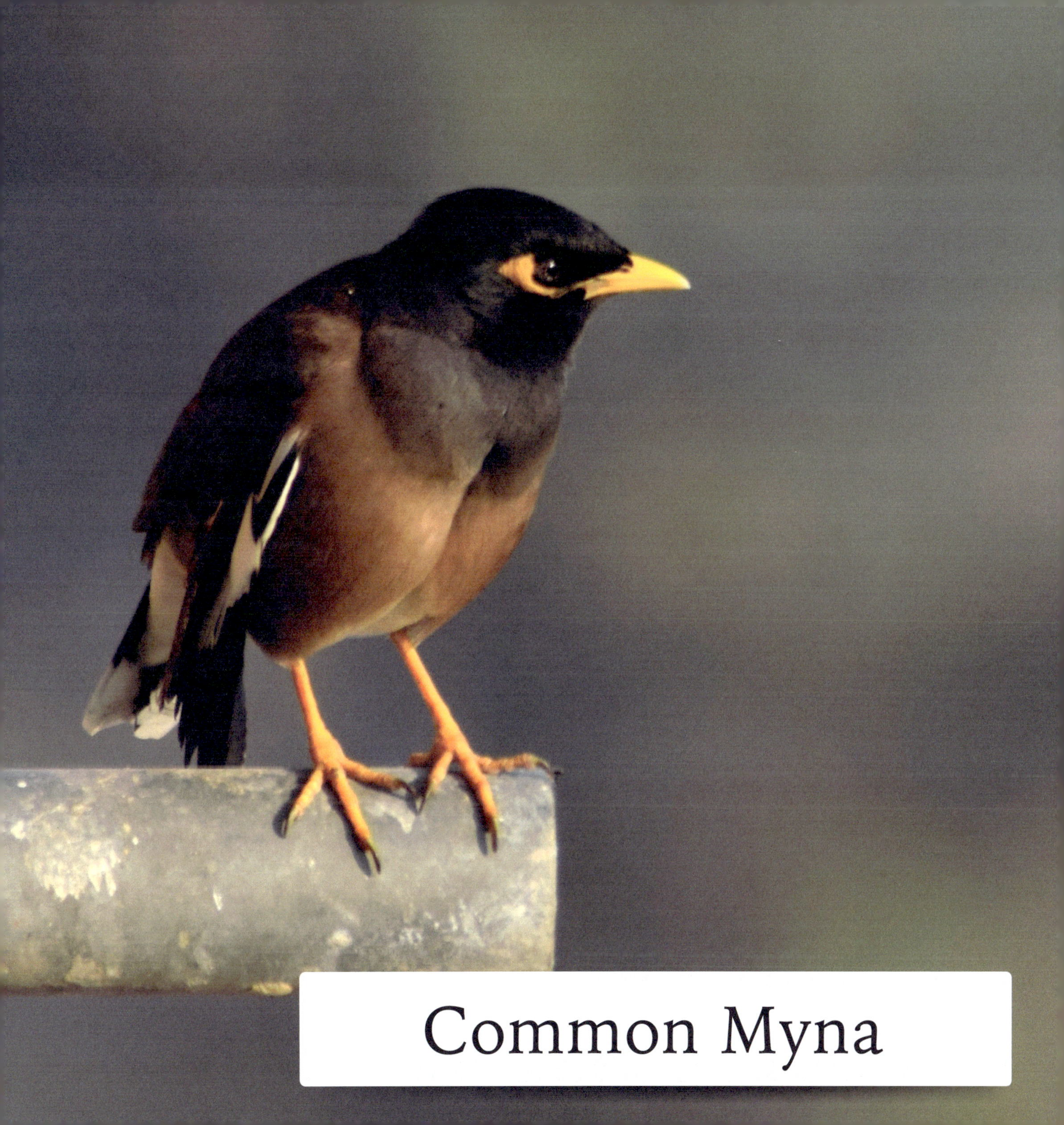

Common Myna

Baby Ducks

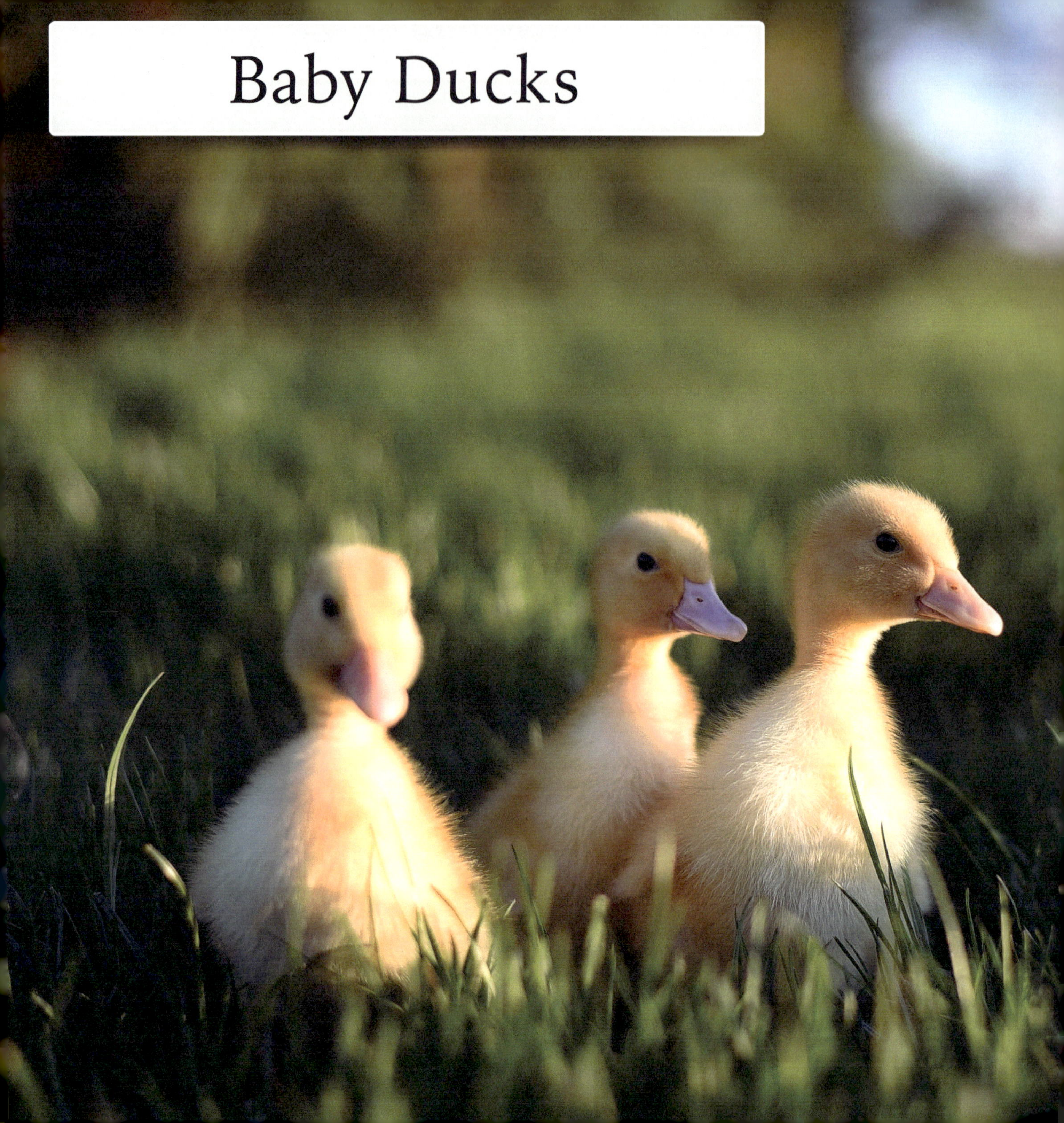

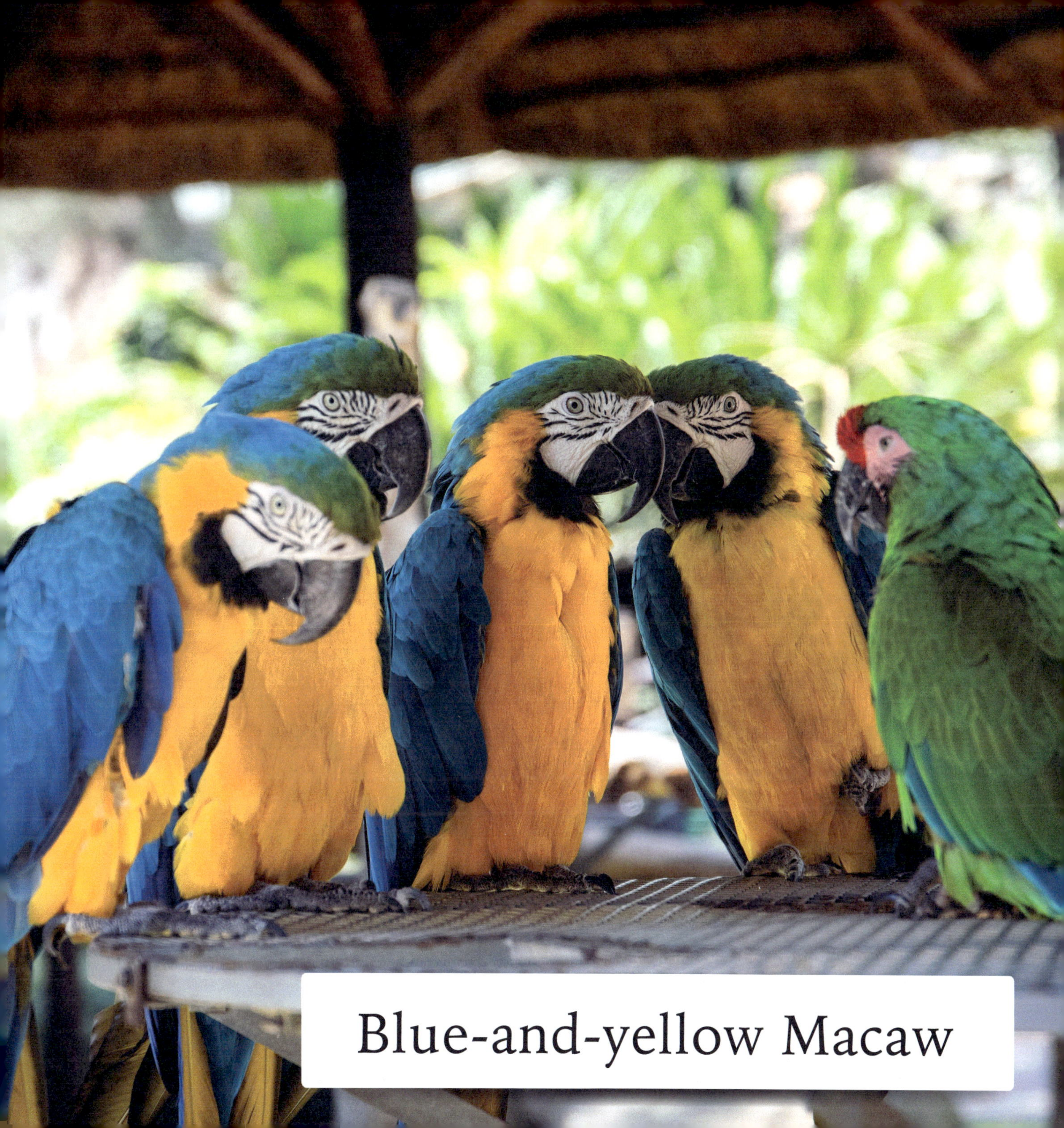

Blue-and-yellow Macaw

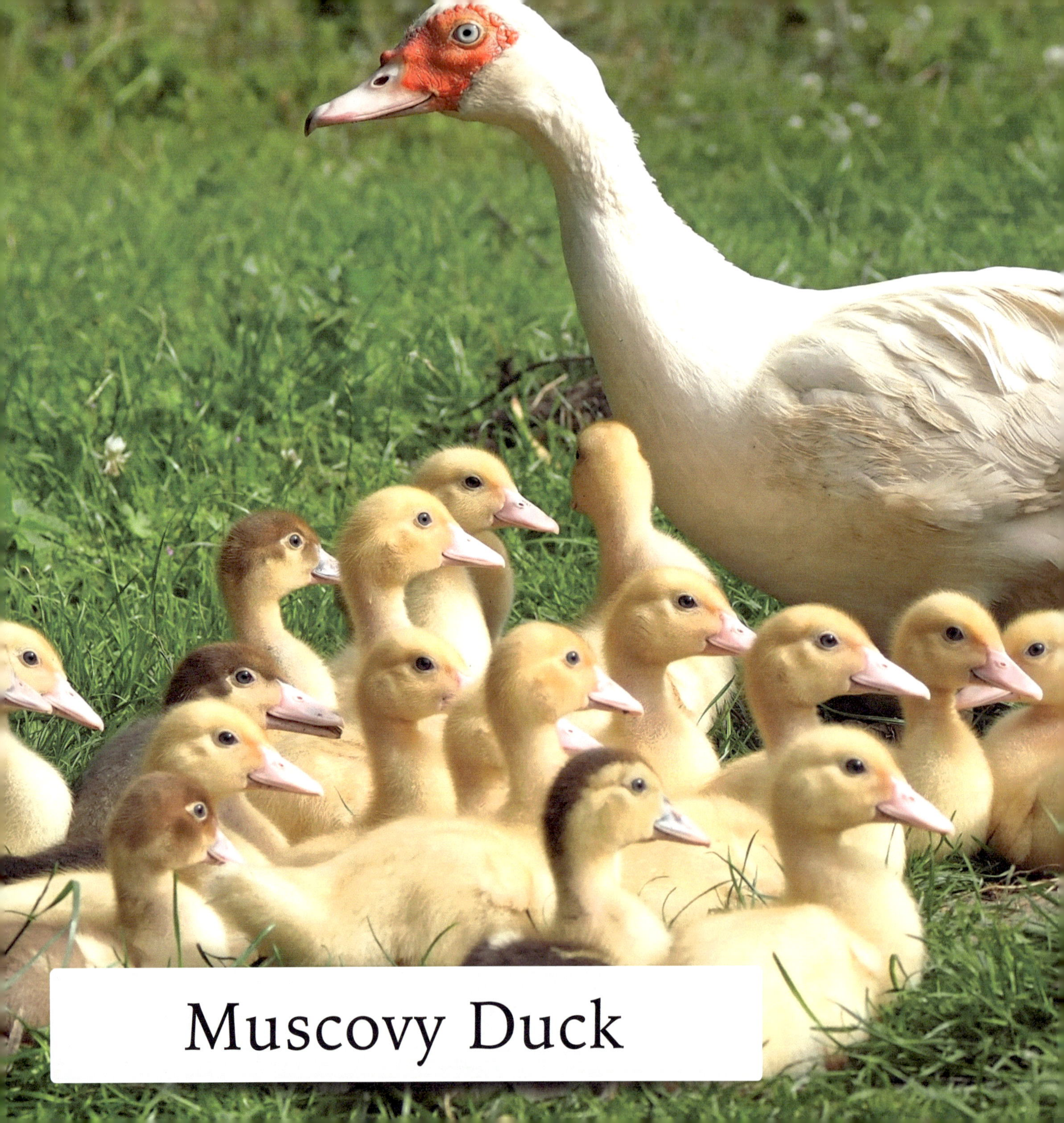

Muscovy Duck

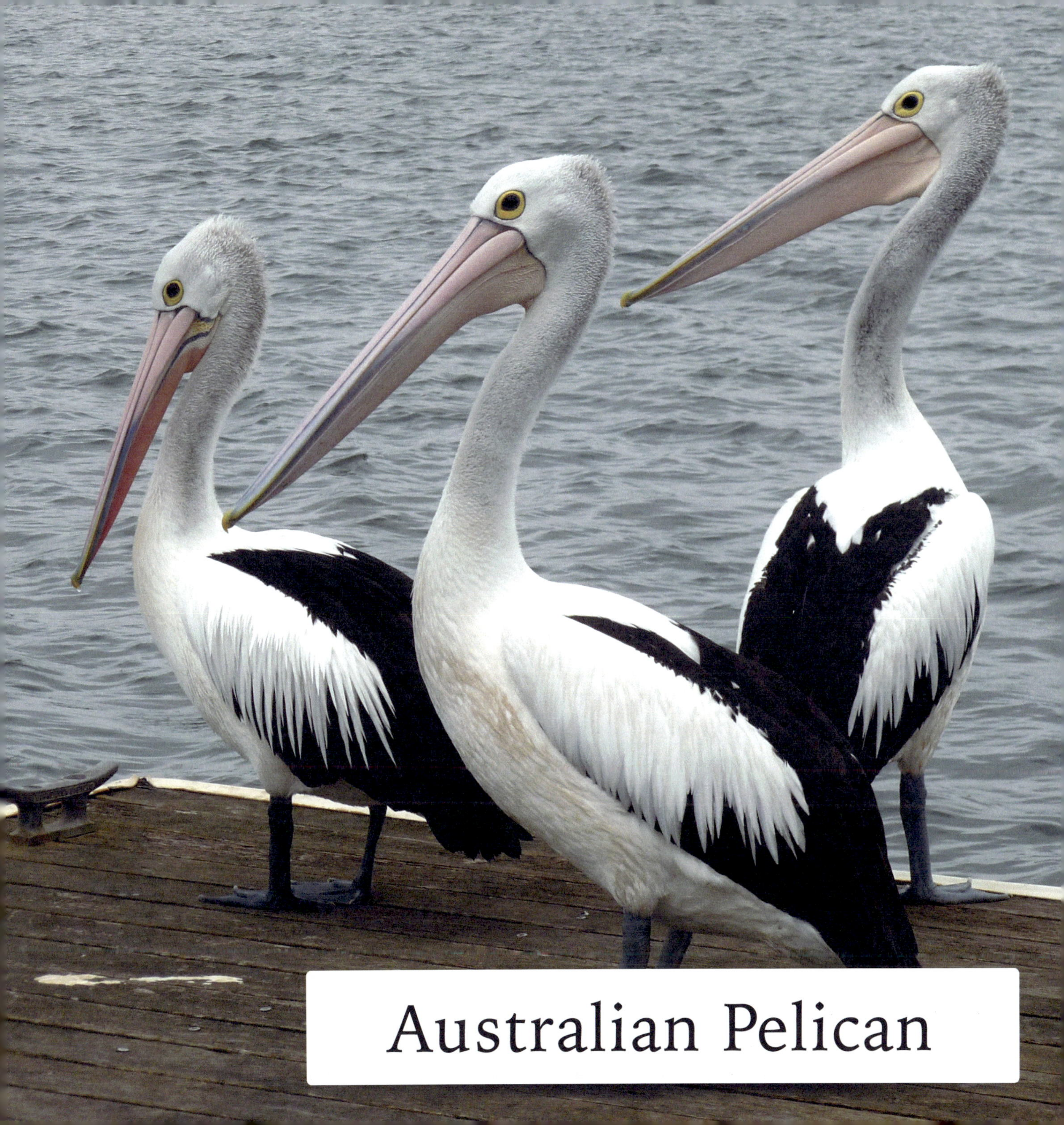

Australian Pelican

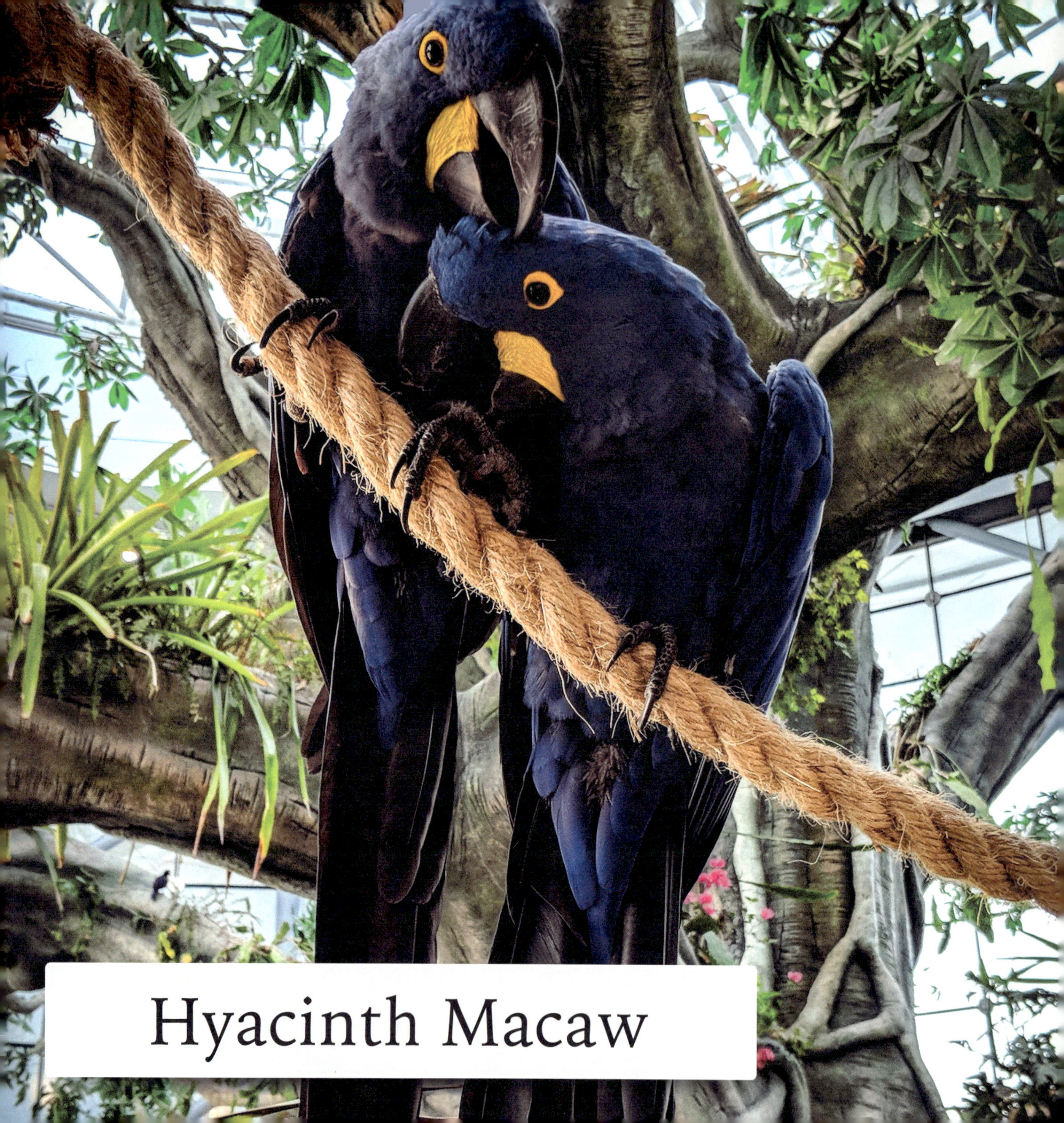

Hyacinth Macaw

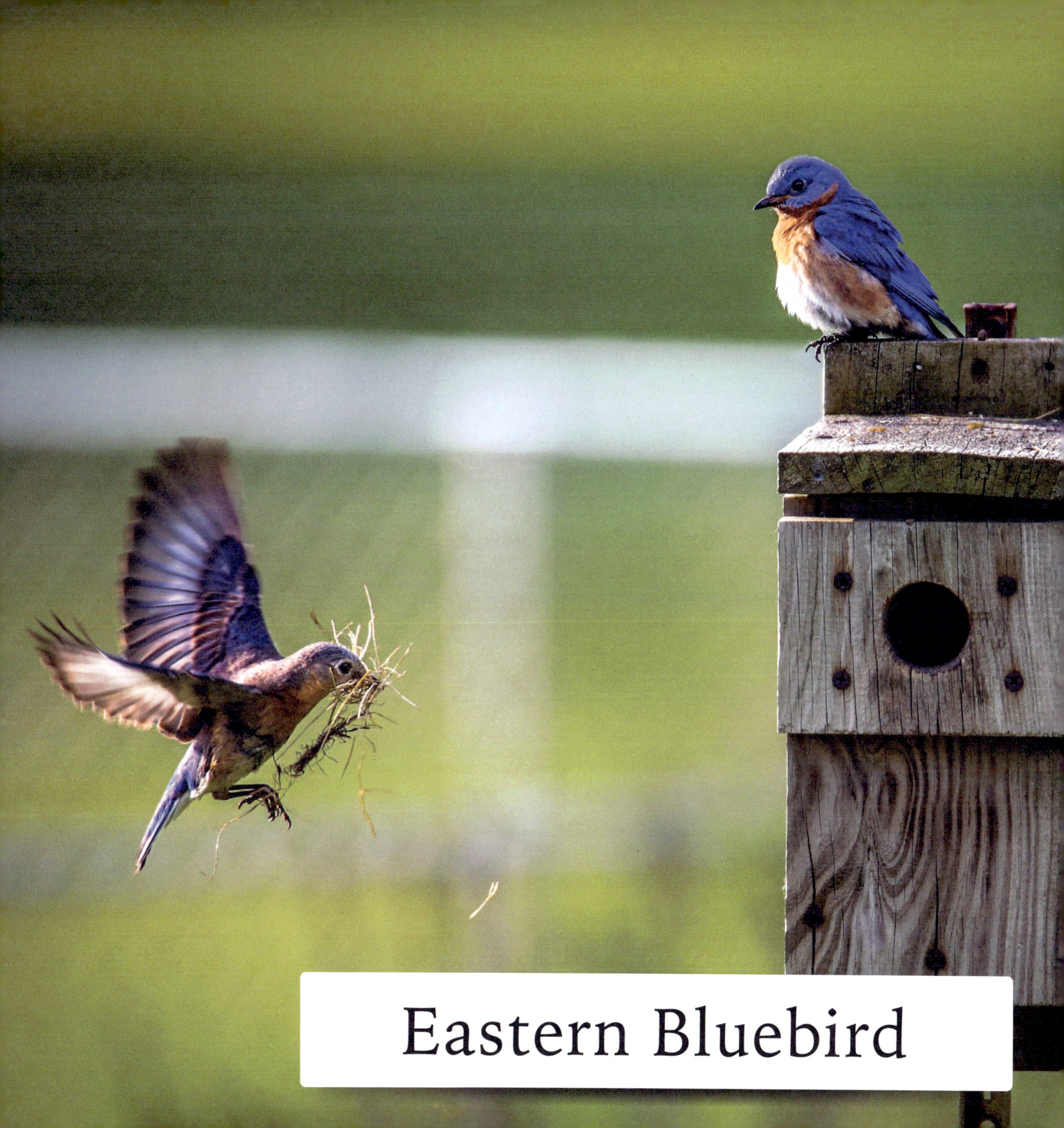

Eastern Bluebird

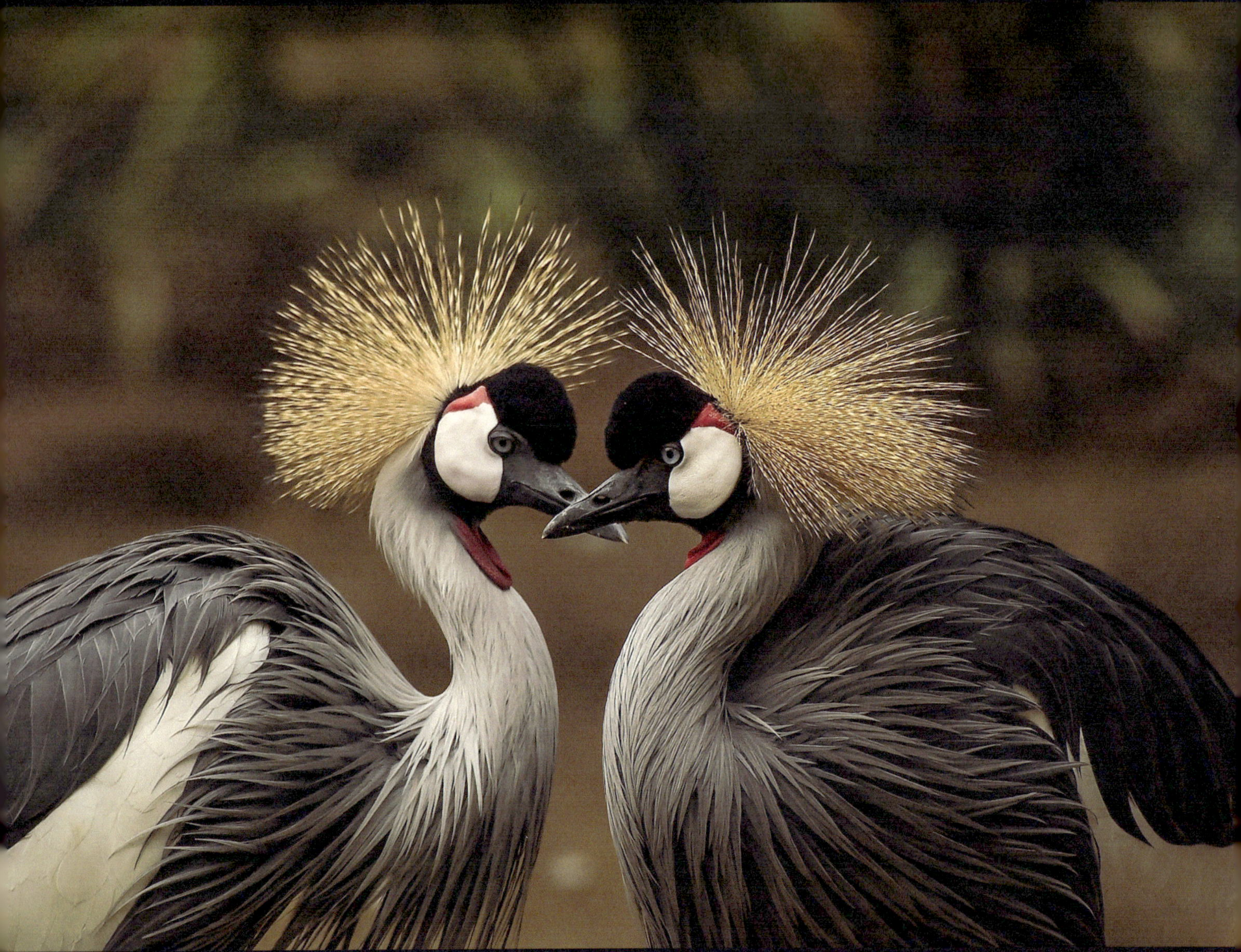

Grey Crowned-Crane

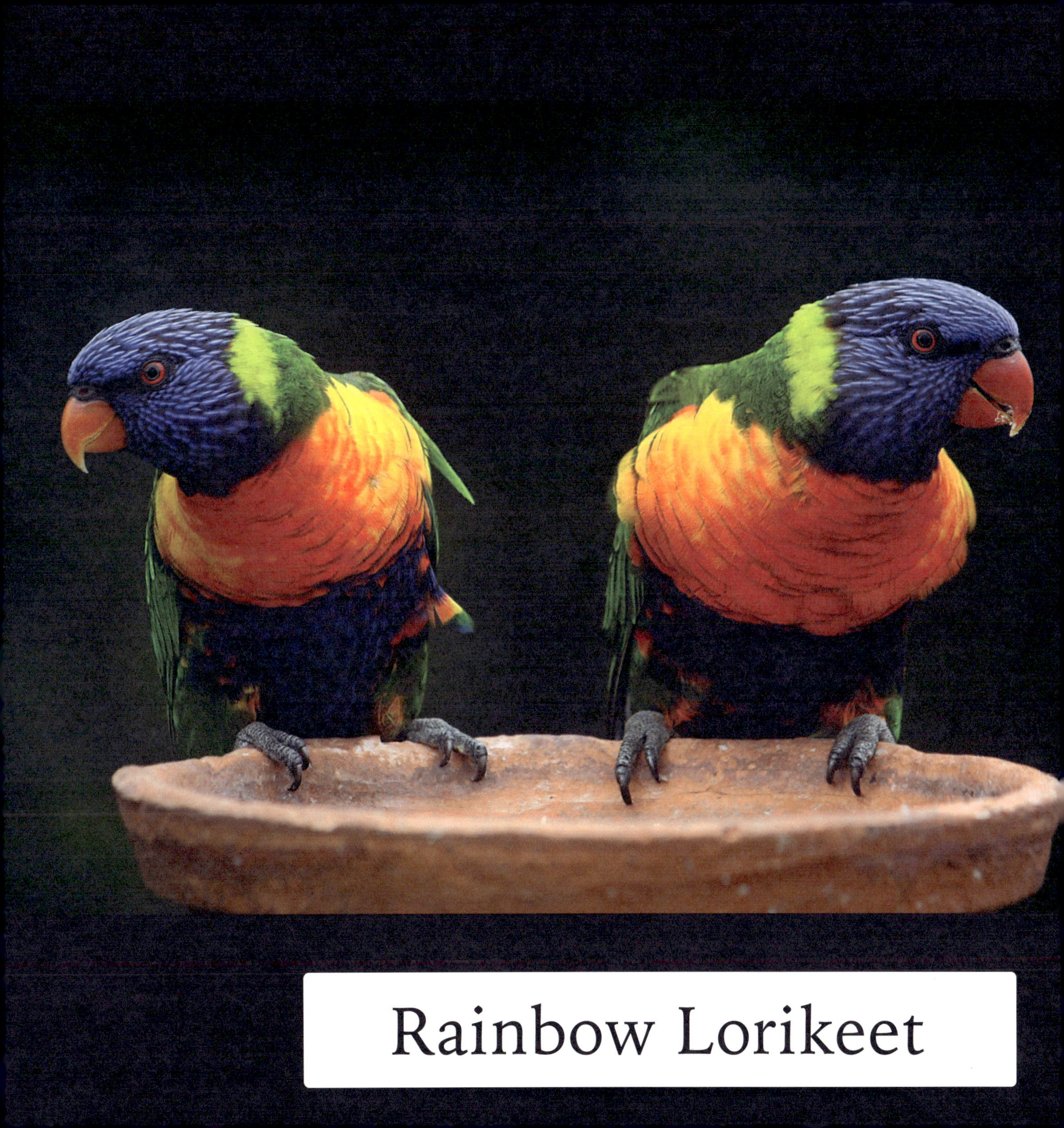

Rainbow Lorikeet

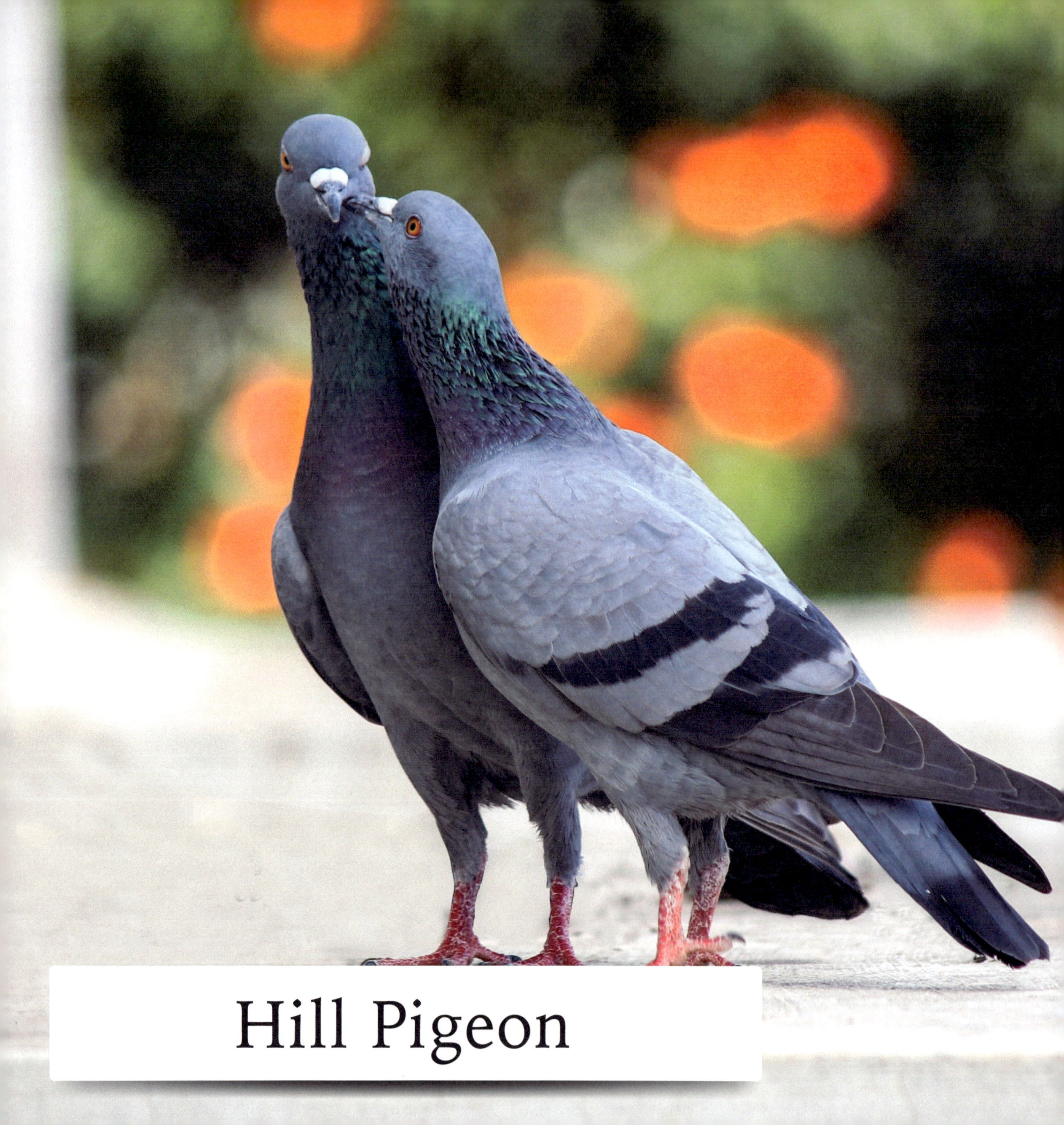

Hill Pigeon

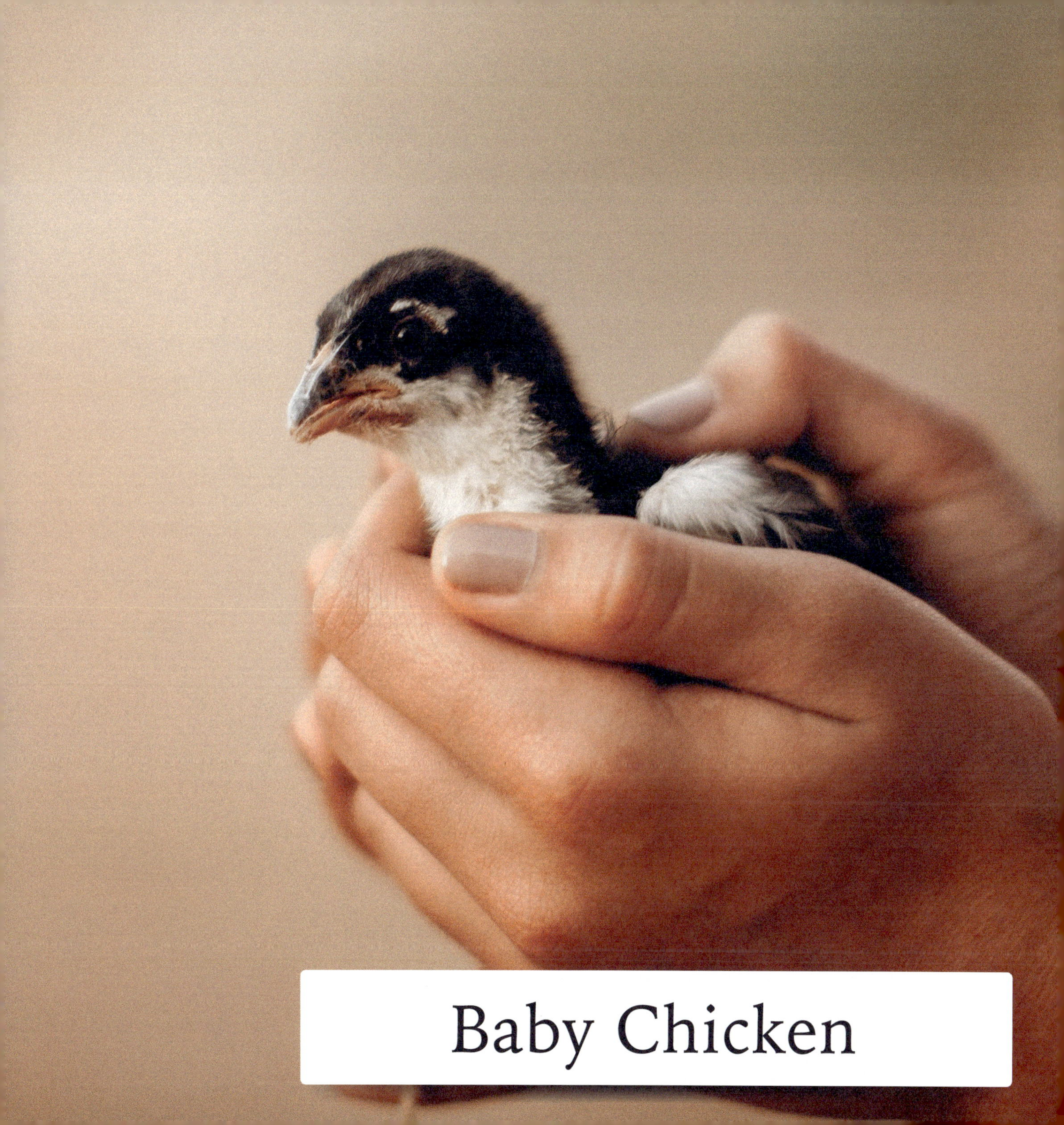

Baby Chicken

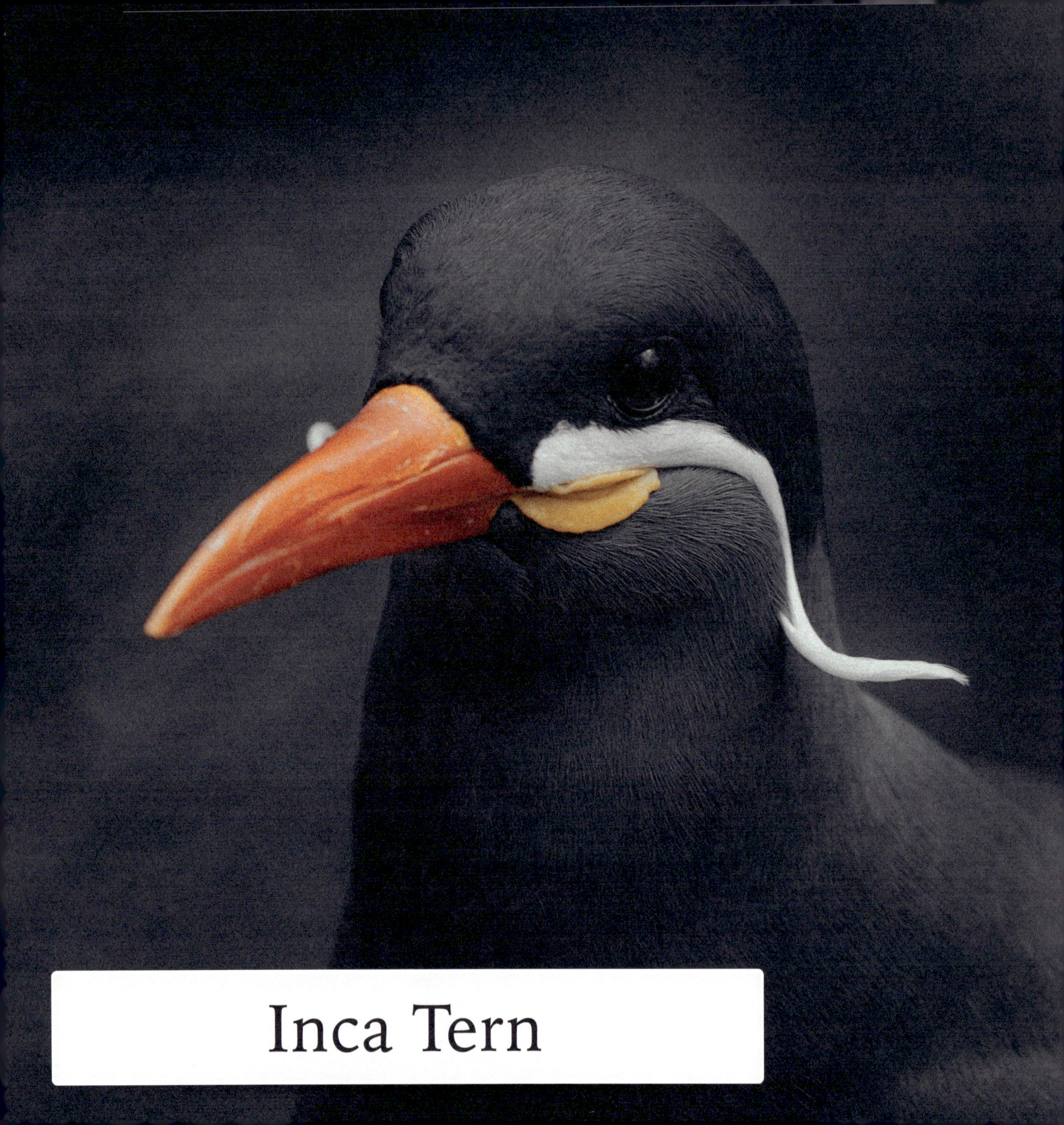

Inca Tern

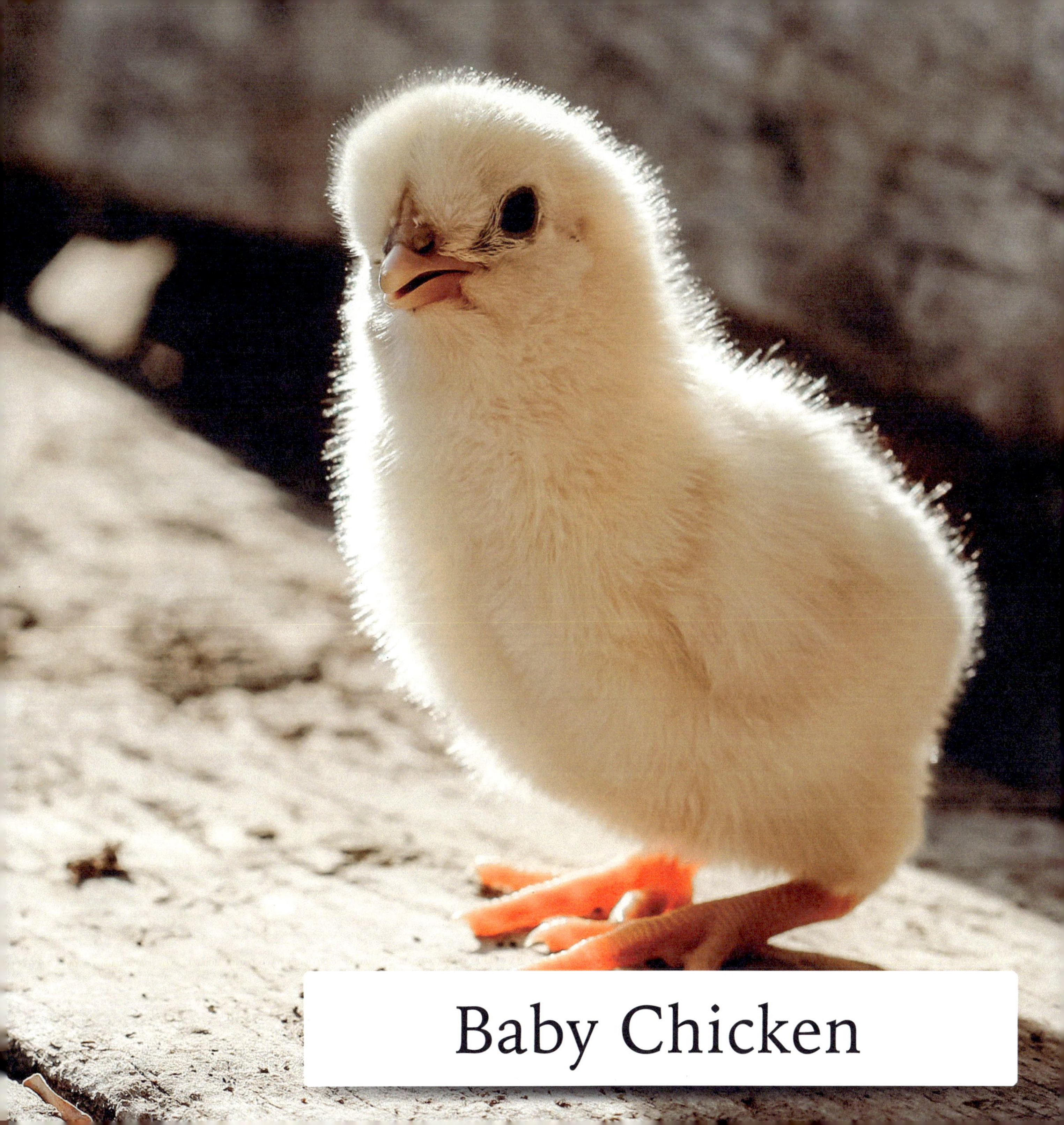

Baby Chicken

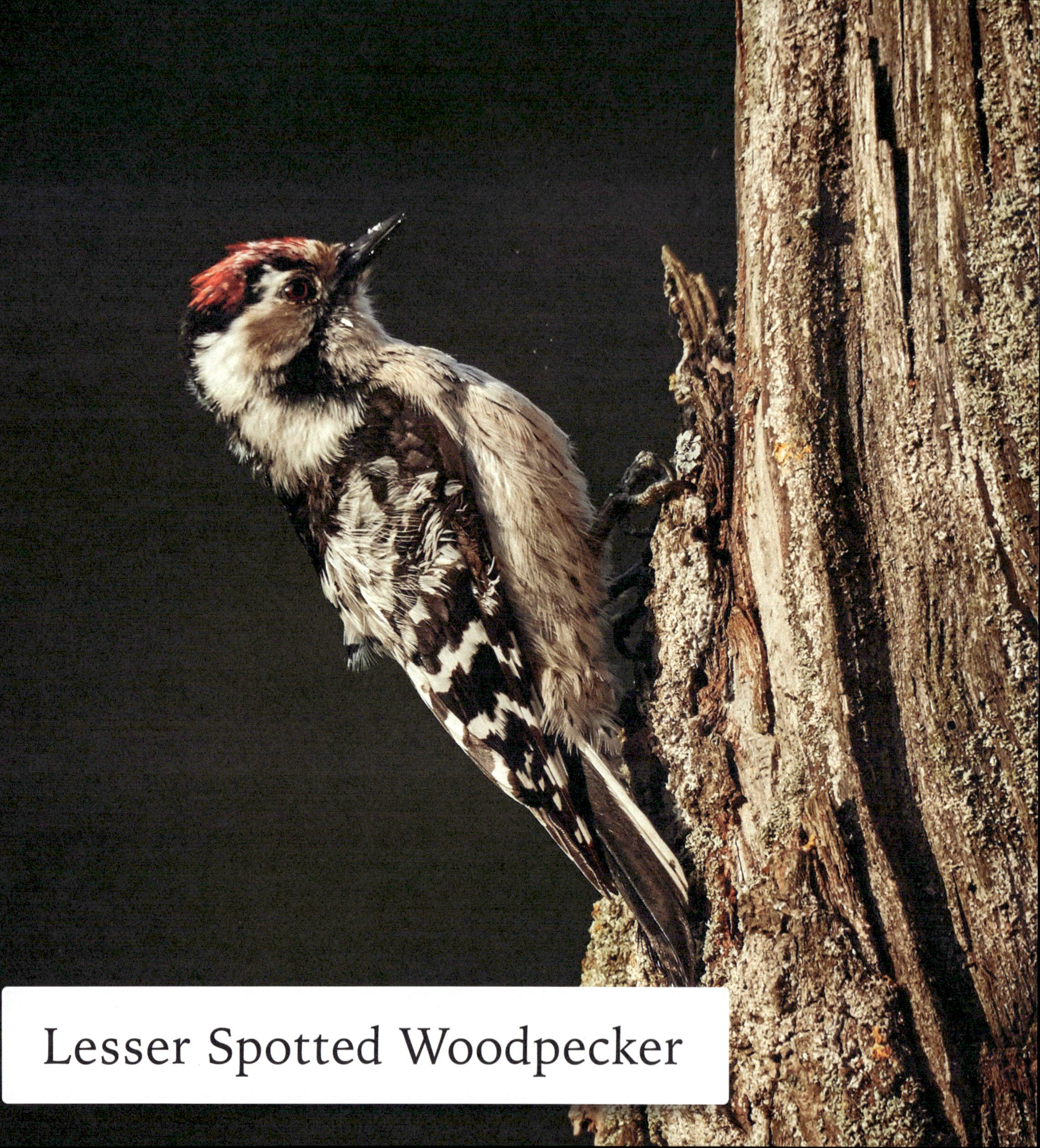

Lesser Spotted Woodpecker

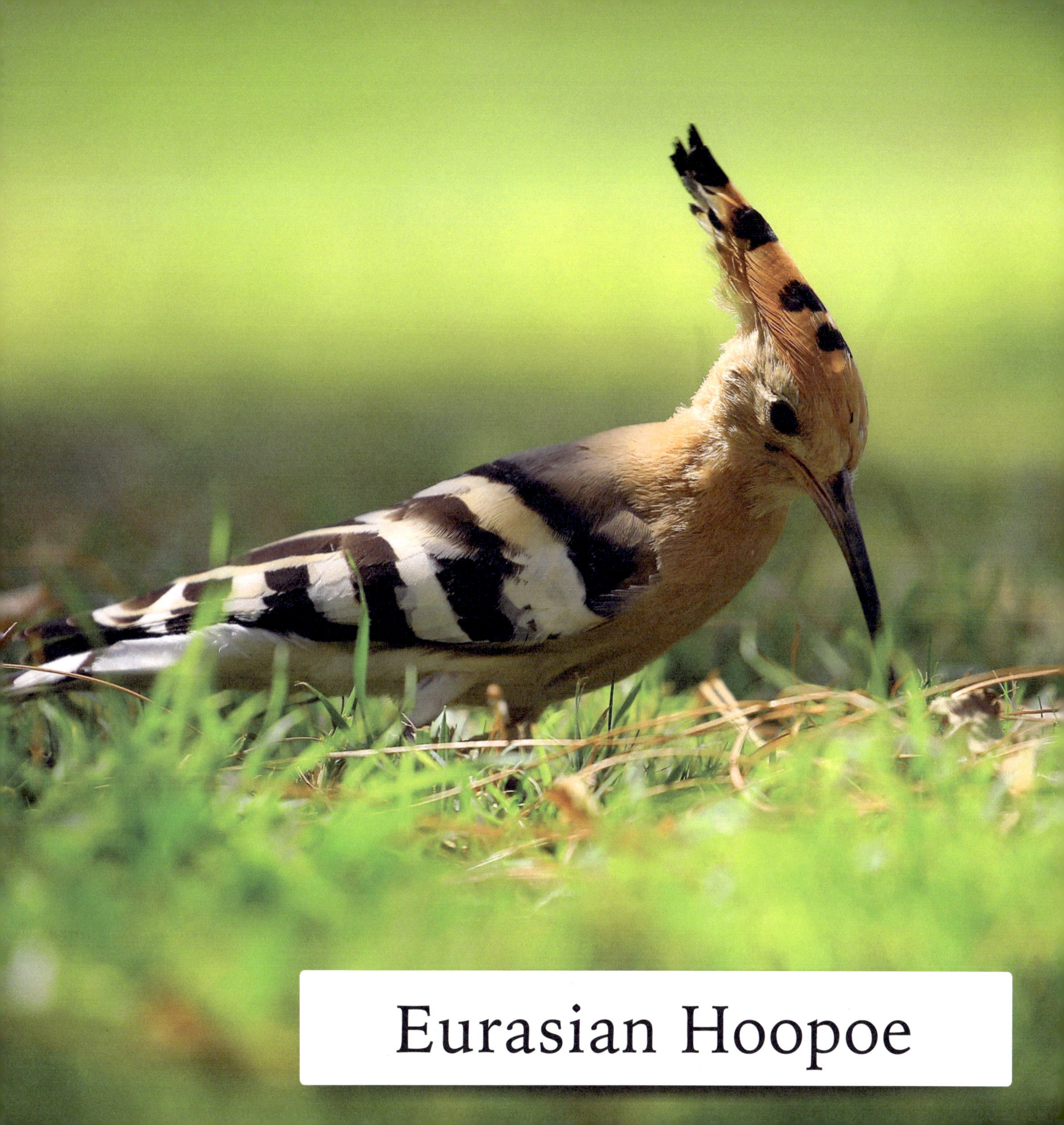

Eurasian Hoopoe

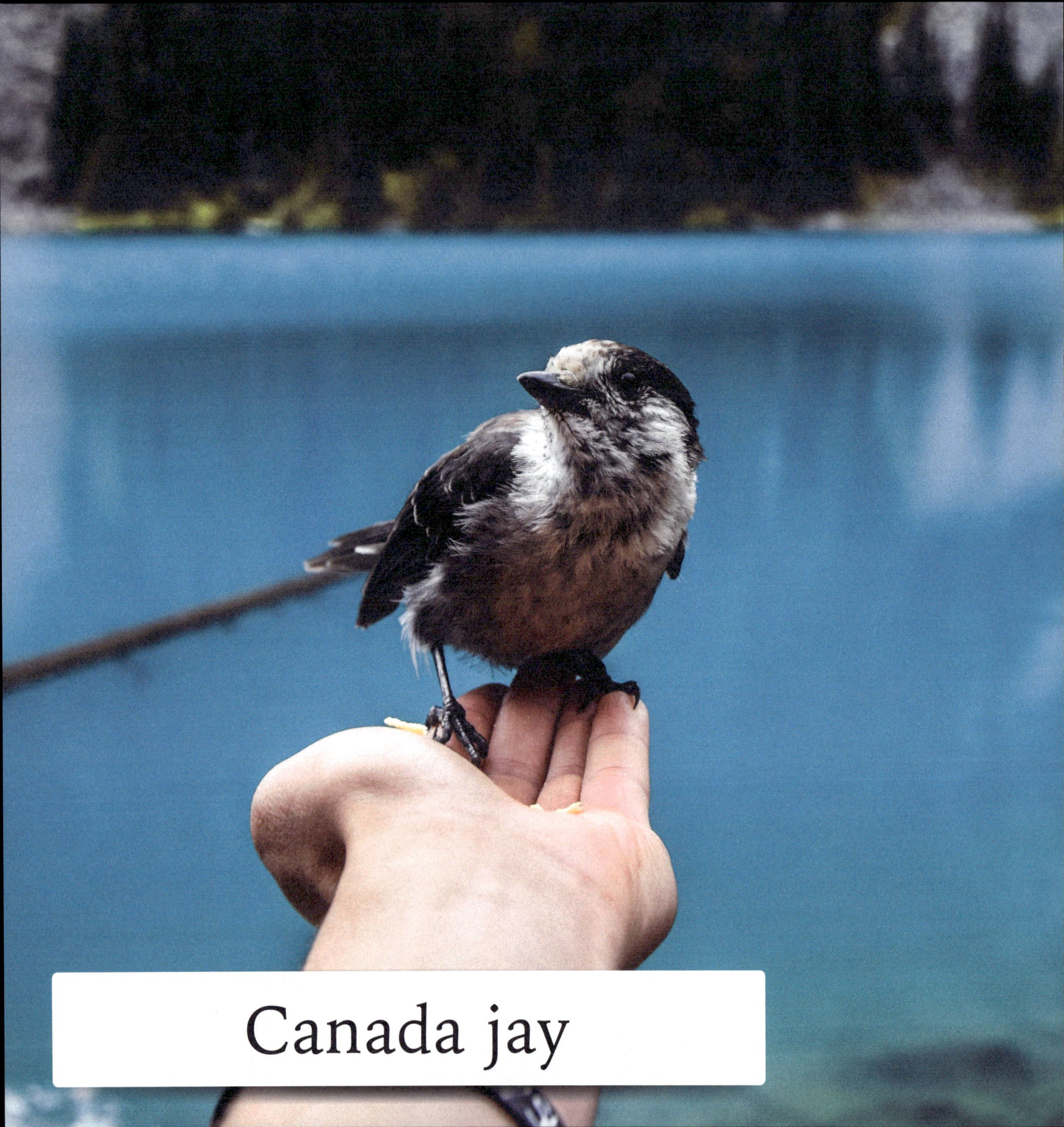
Canada jay

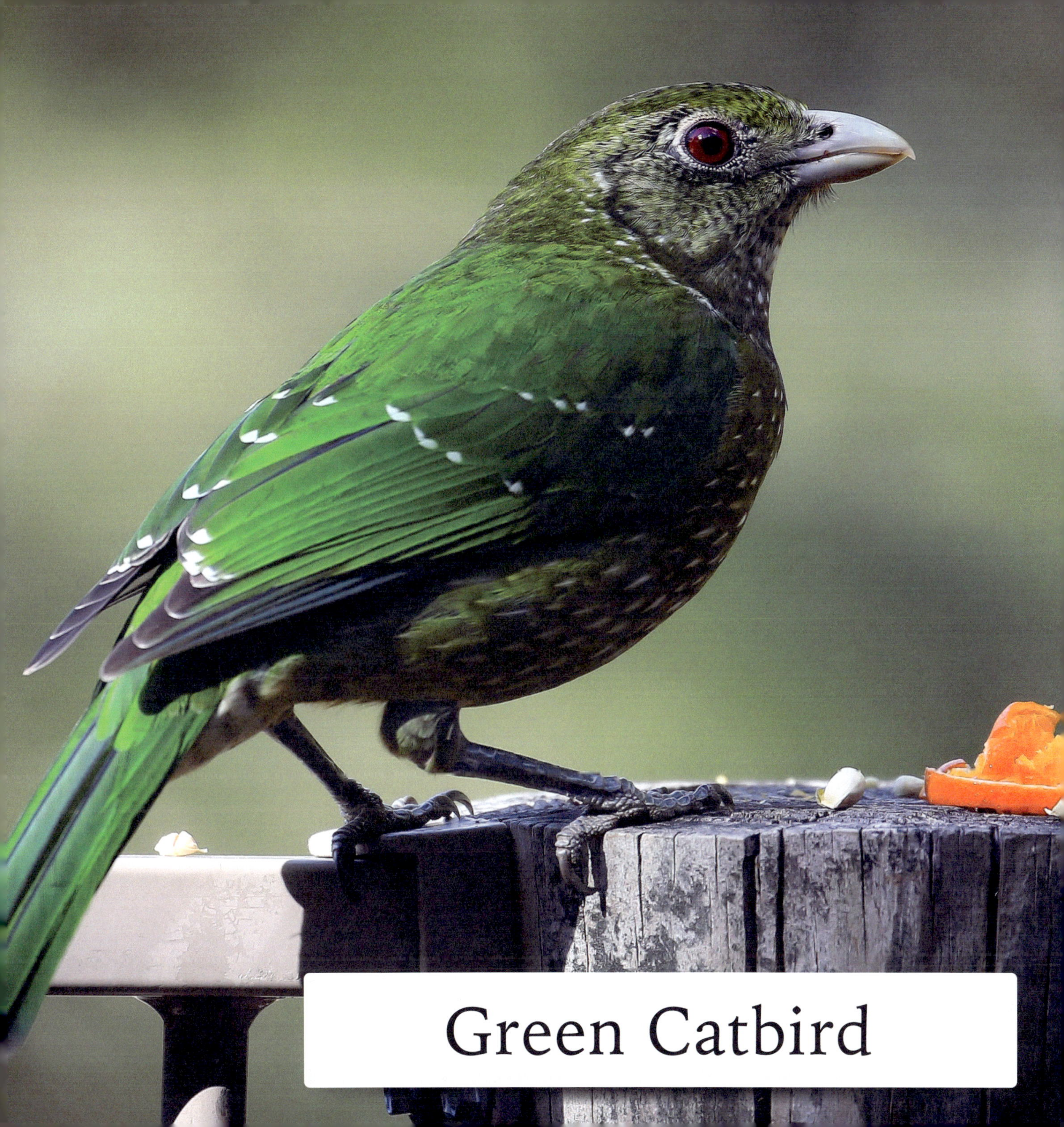

Green Catbird

Bank Myna

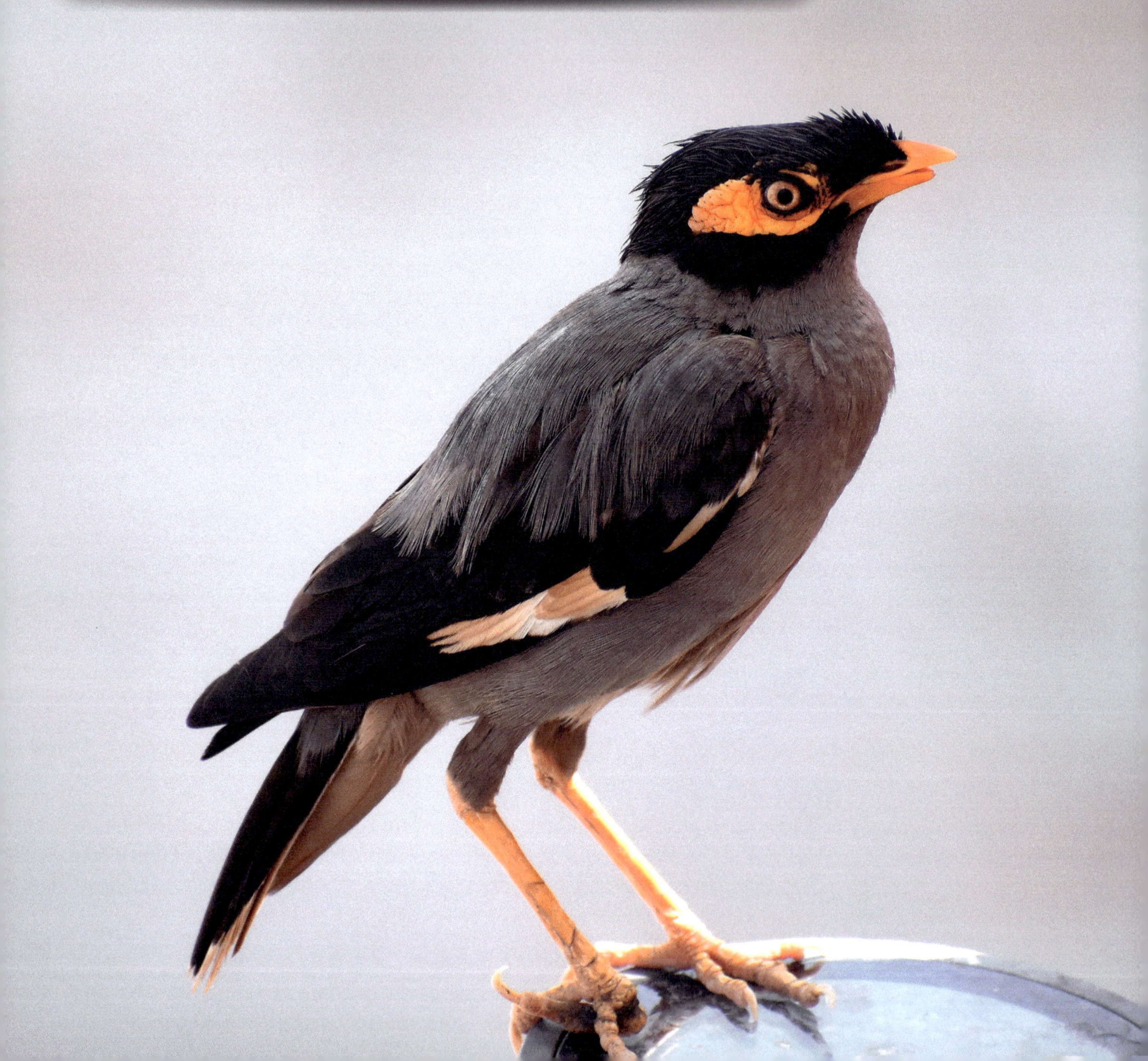

Rock Pigeon

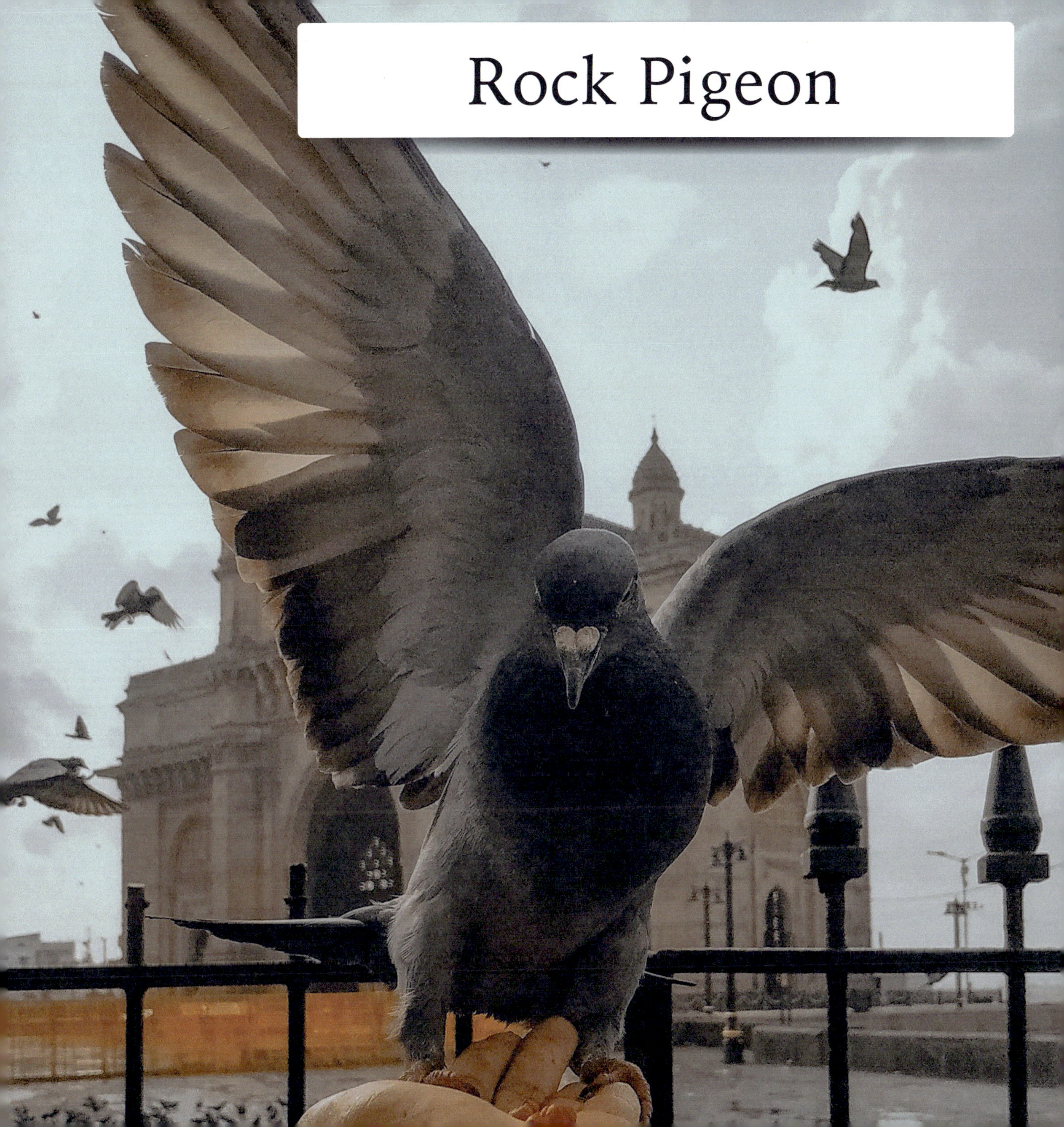

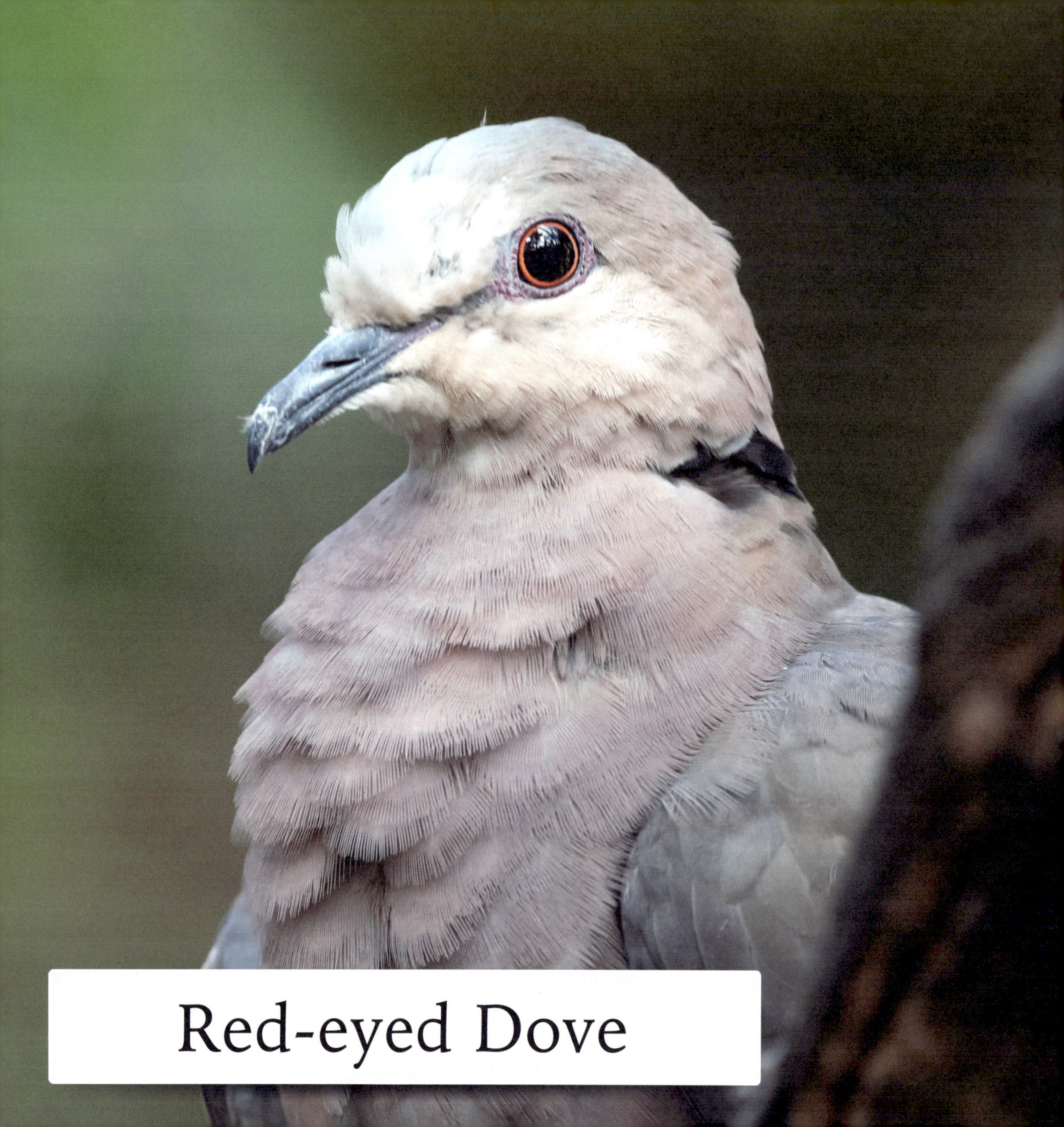

Red-eyed Dove

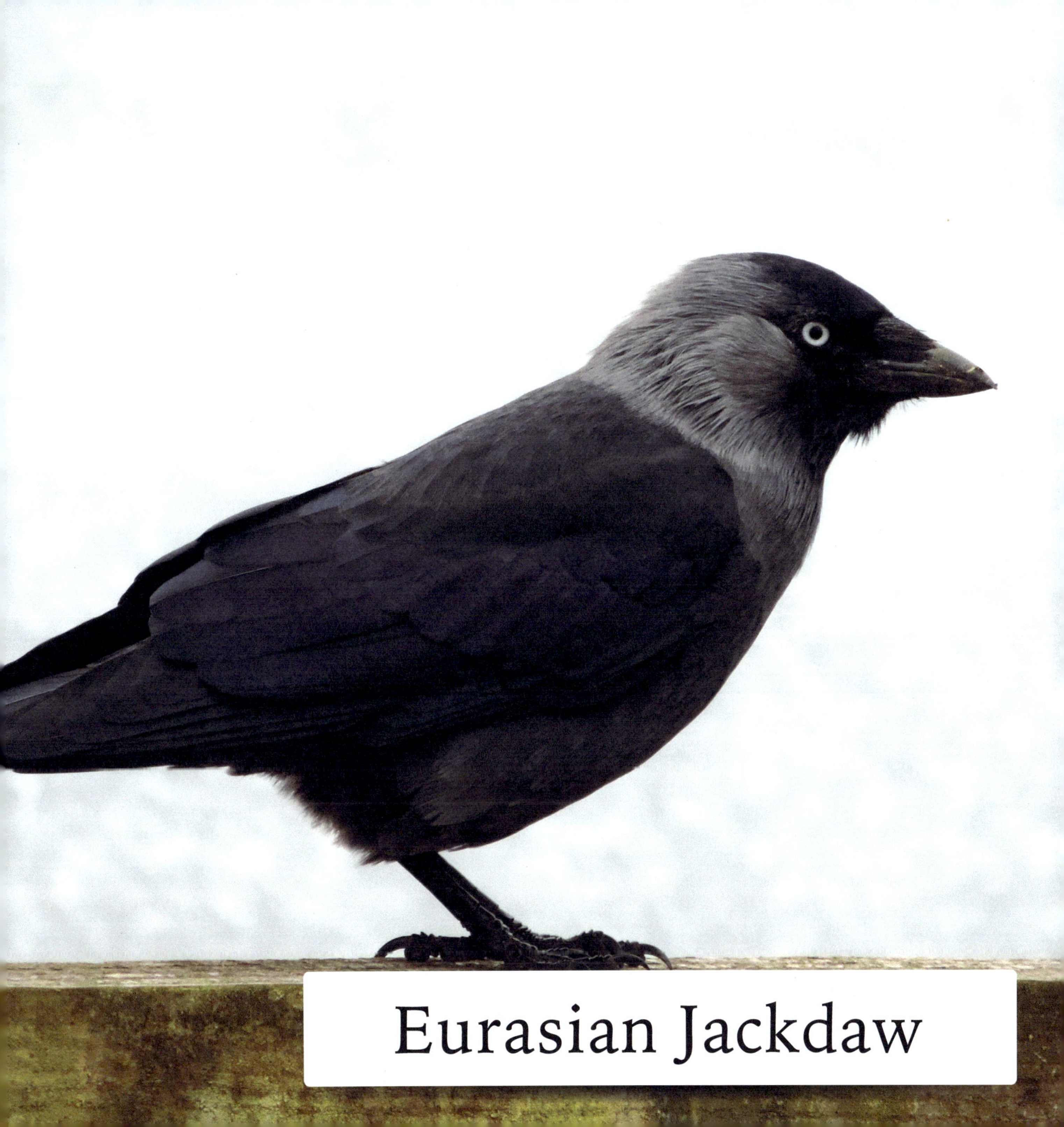

Eurasian Jackdaw

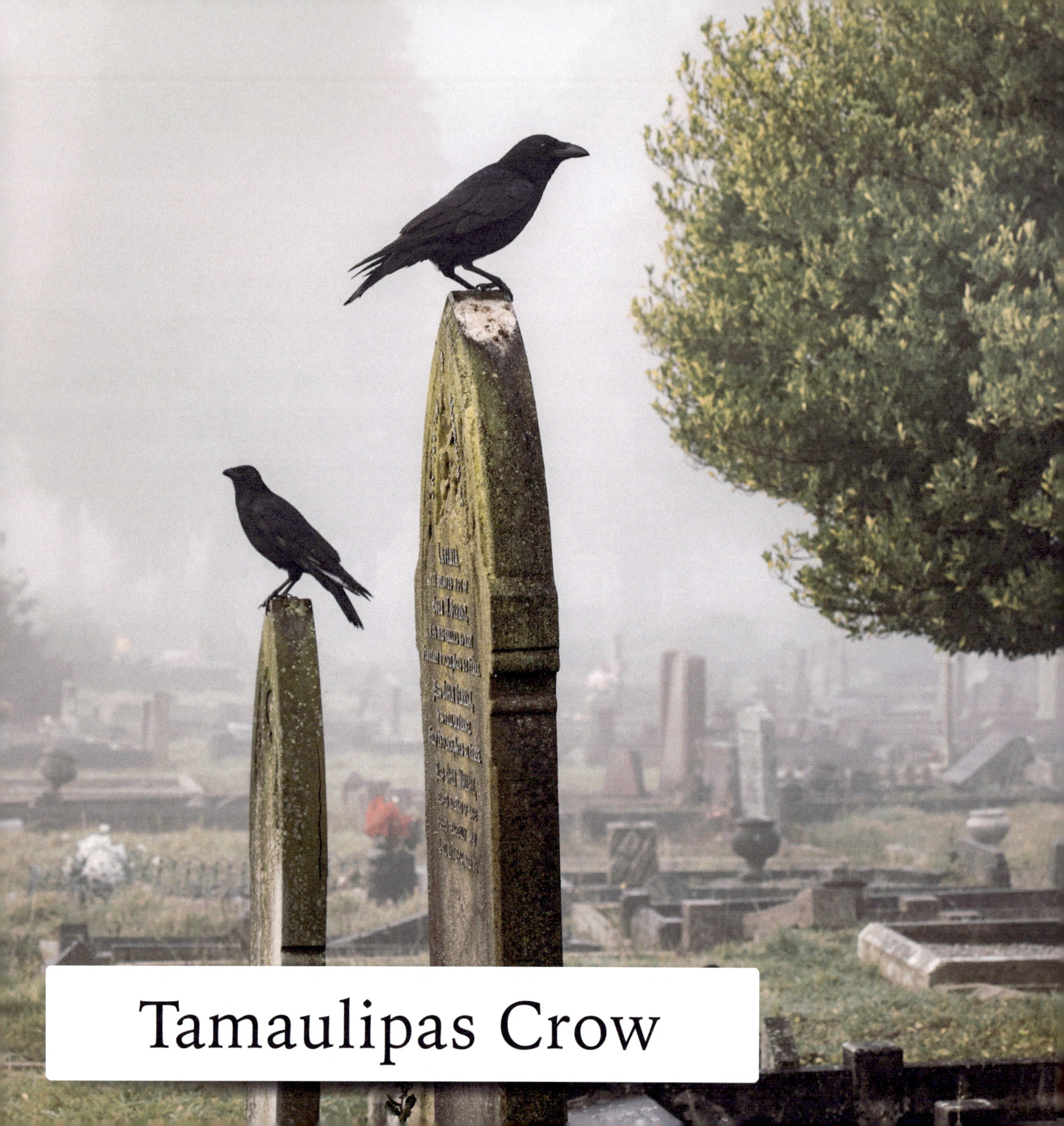

Tamaulipas Crow

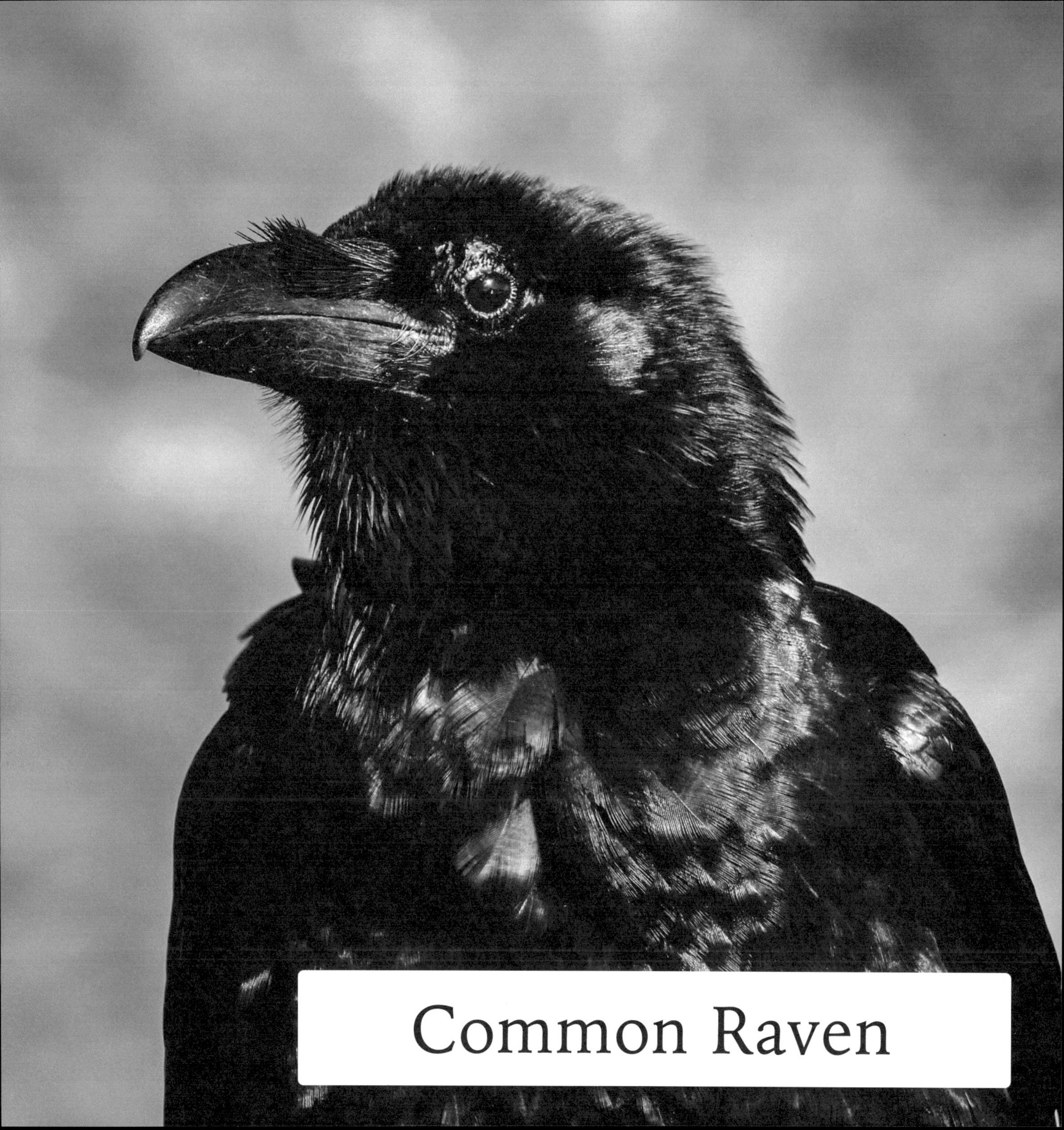

Common Raven

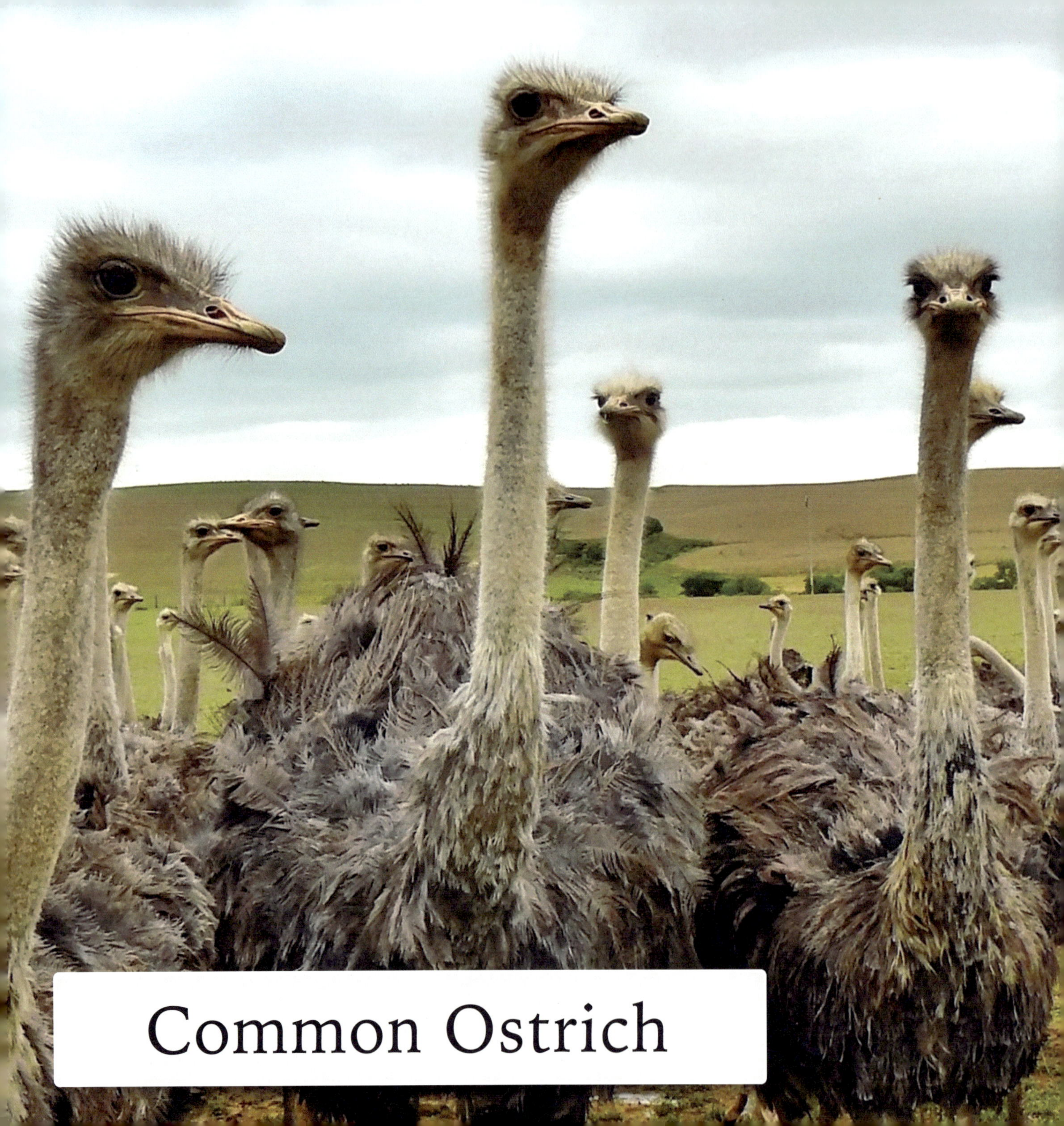

Common Ostrich

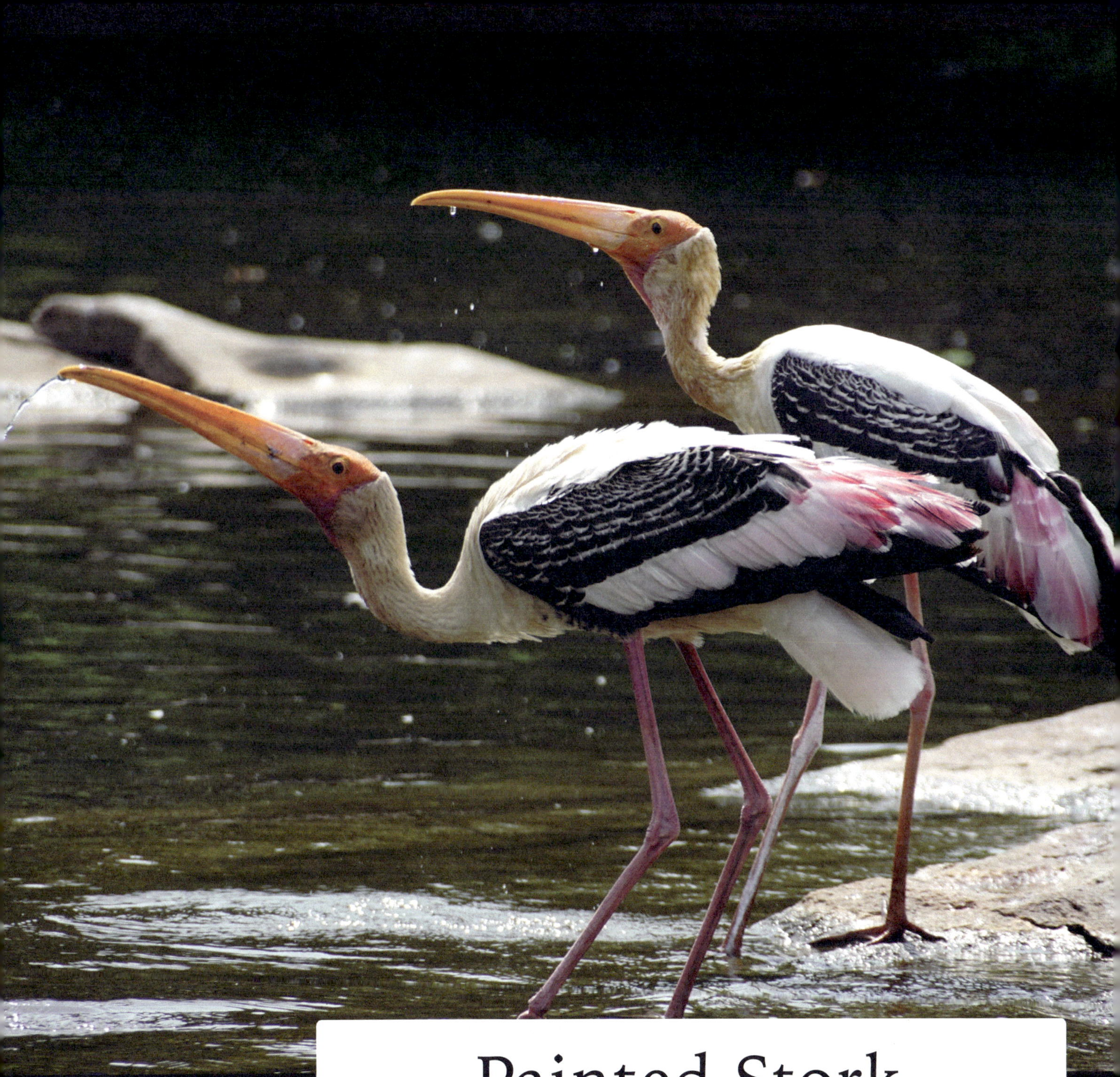

Painted Stork

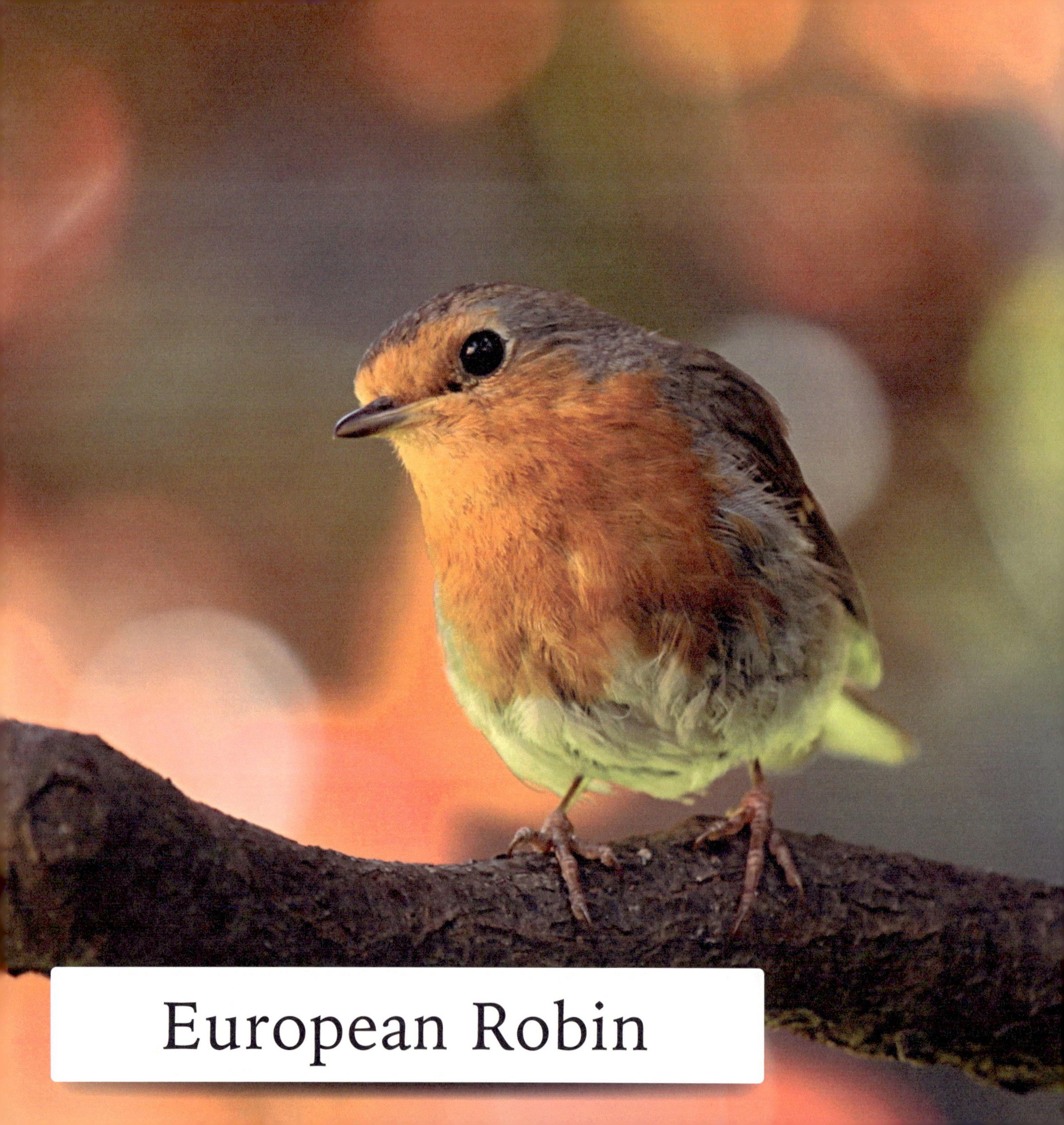

European Robin

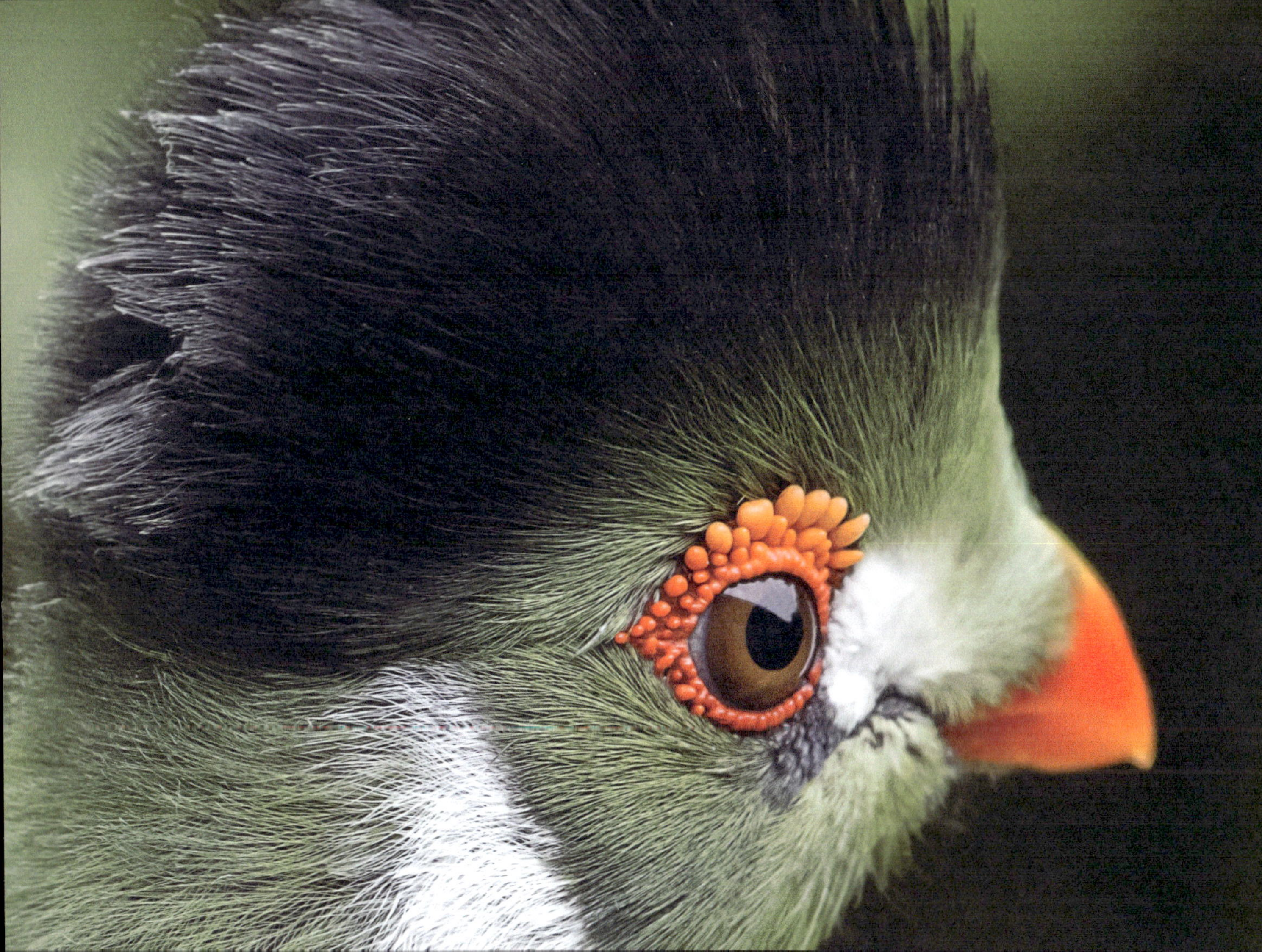

Guinea Turaco

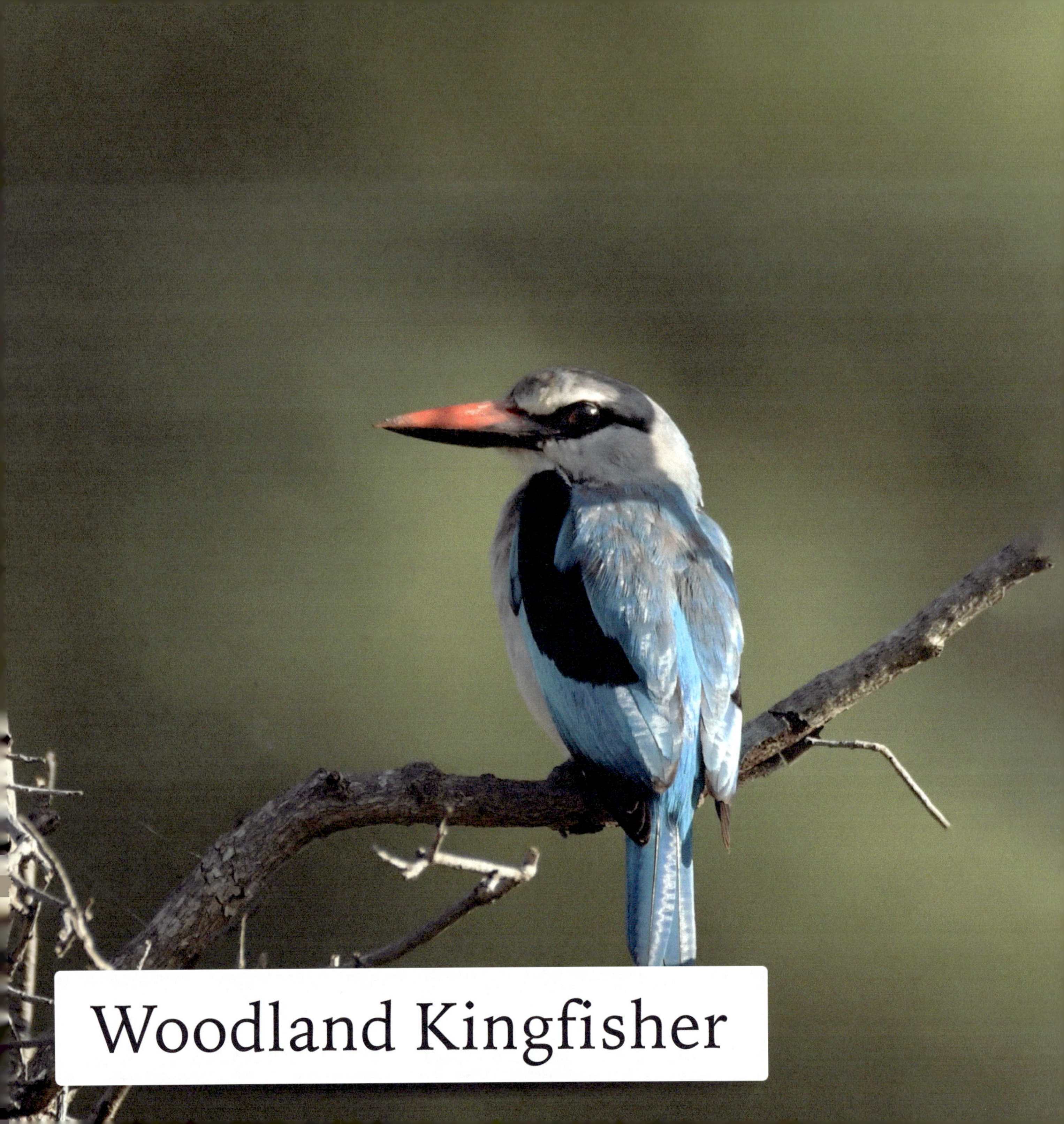

Woodland Kingfisher

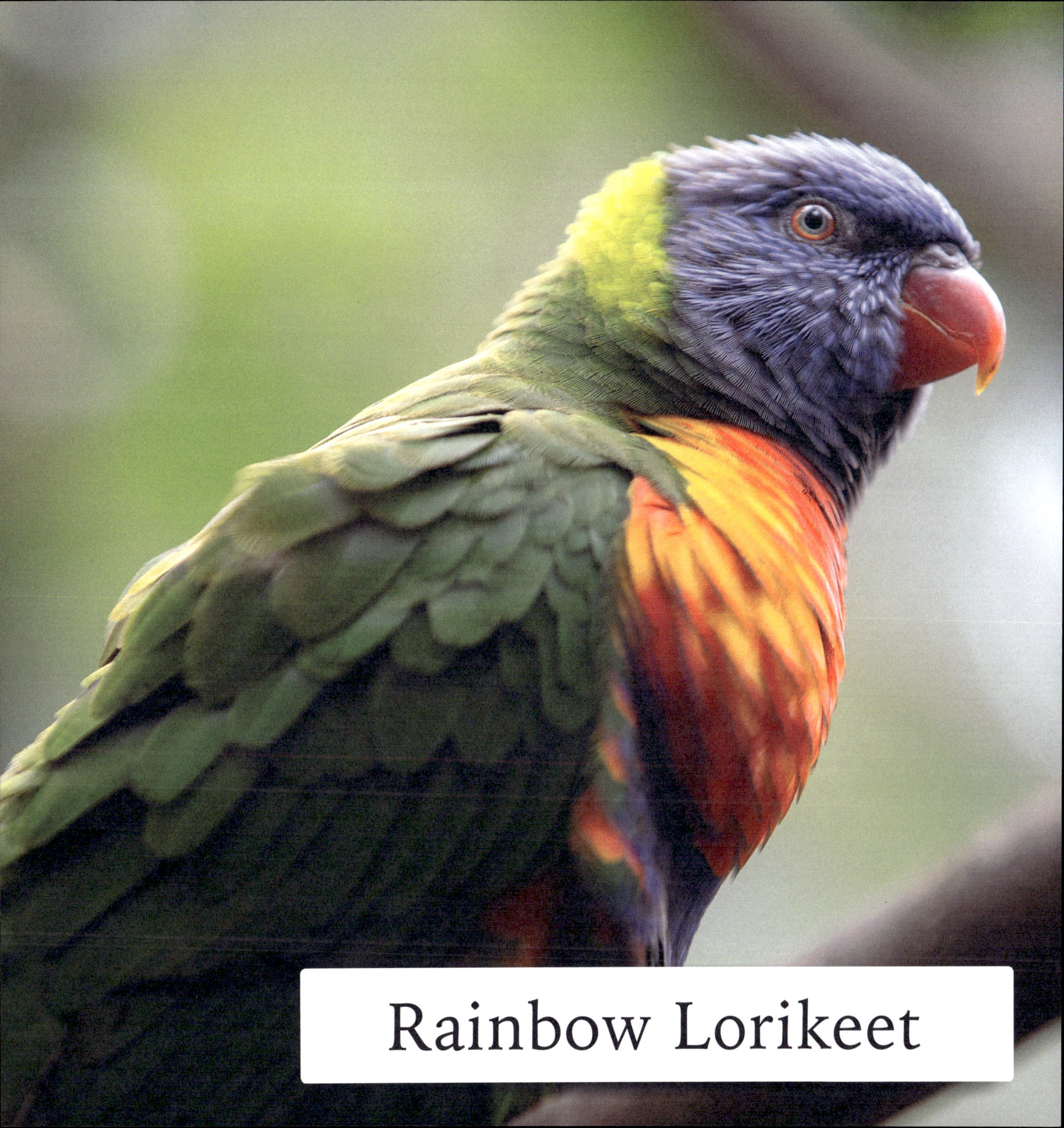

Rainbow Lorikeet

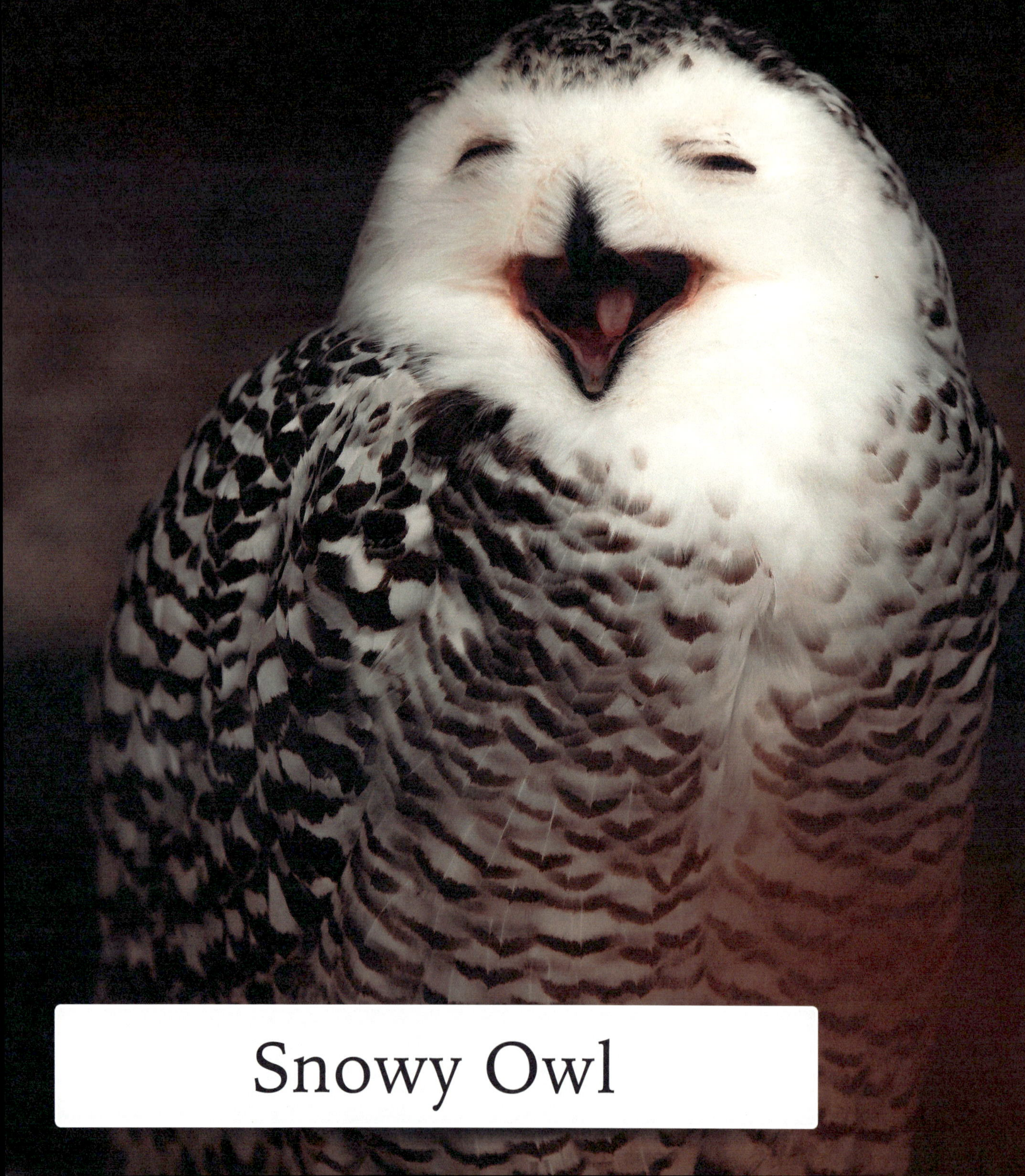

Snowy Owl

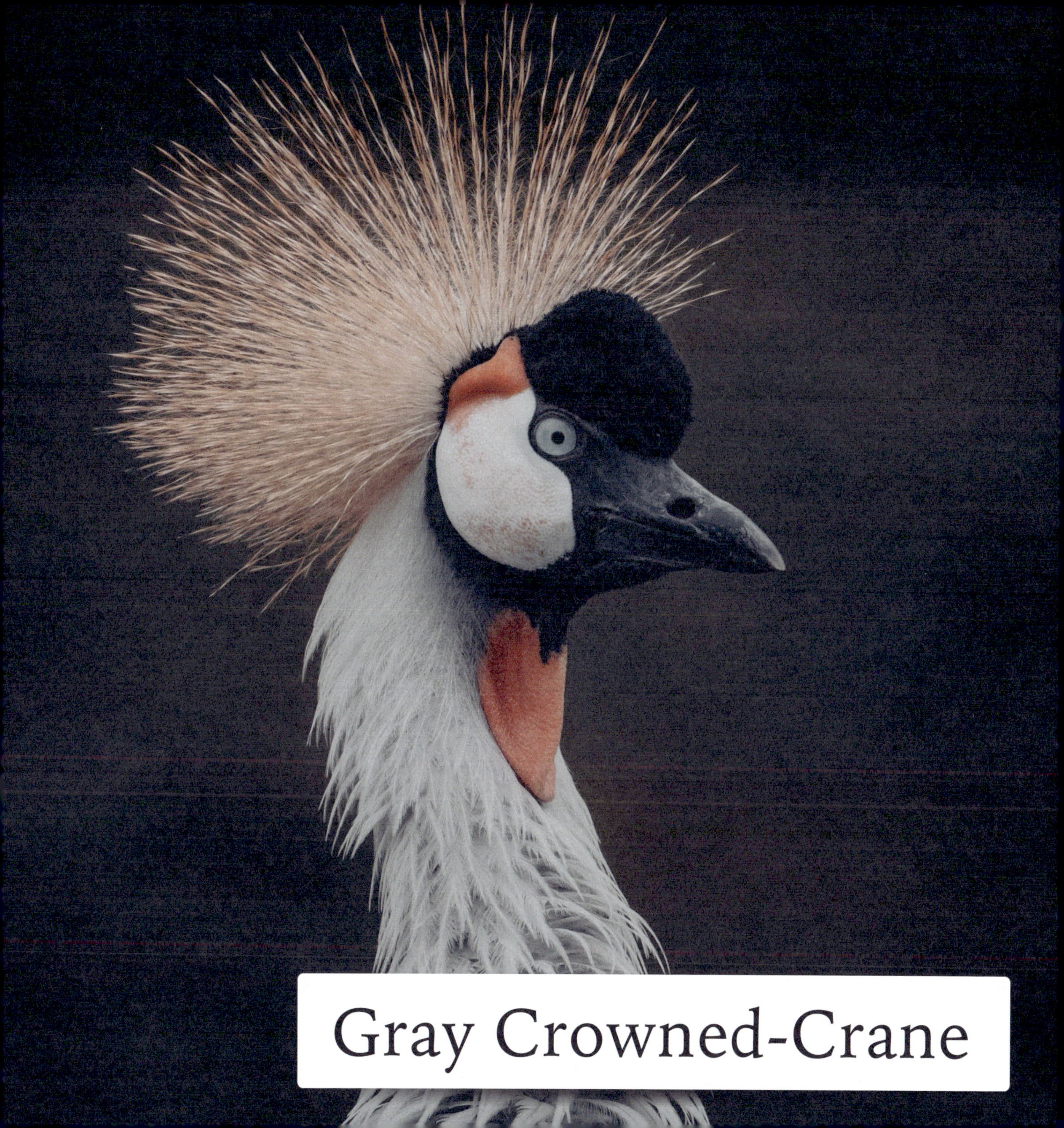

Gray Crowned-Crane

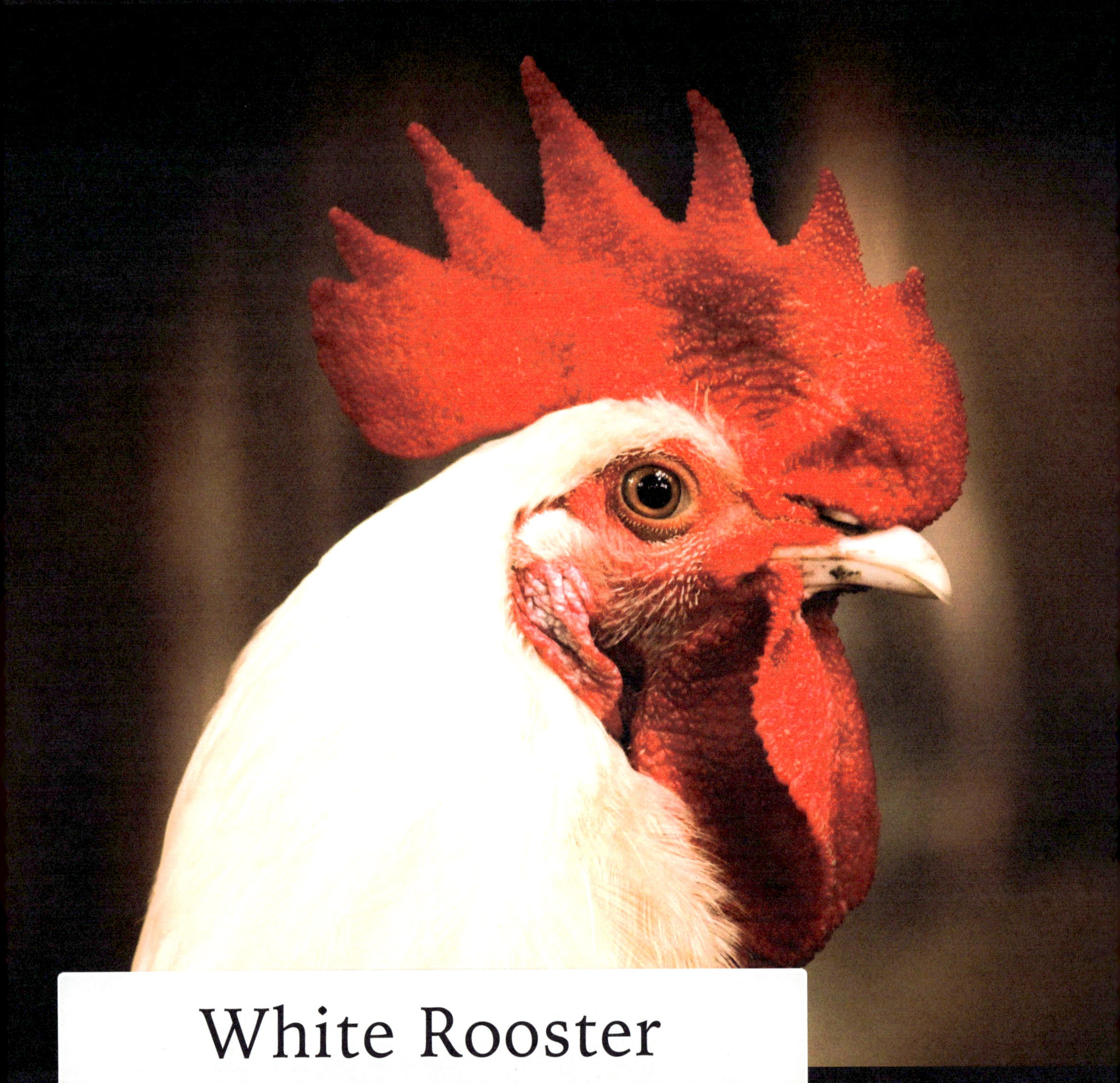

White Rooster

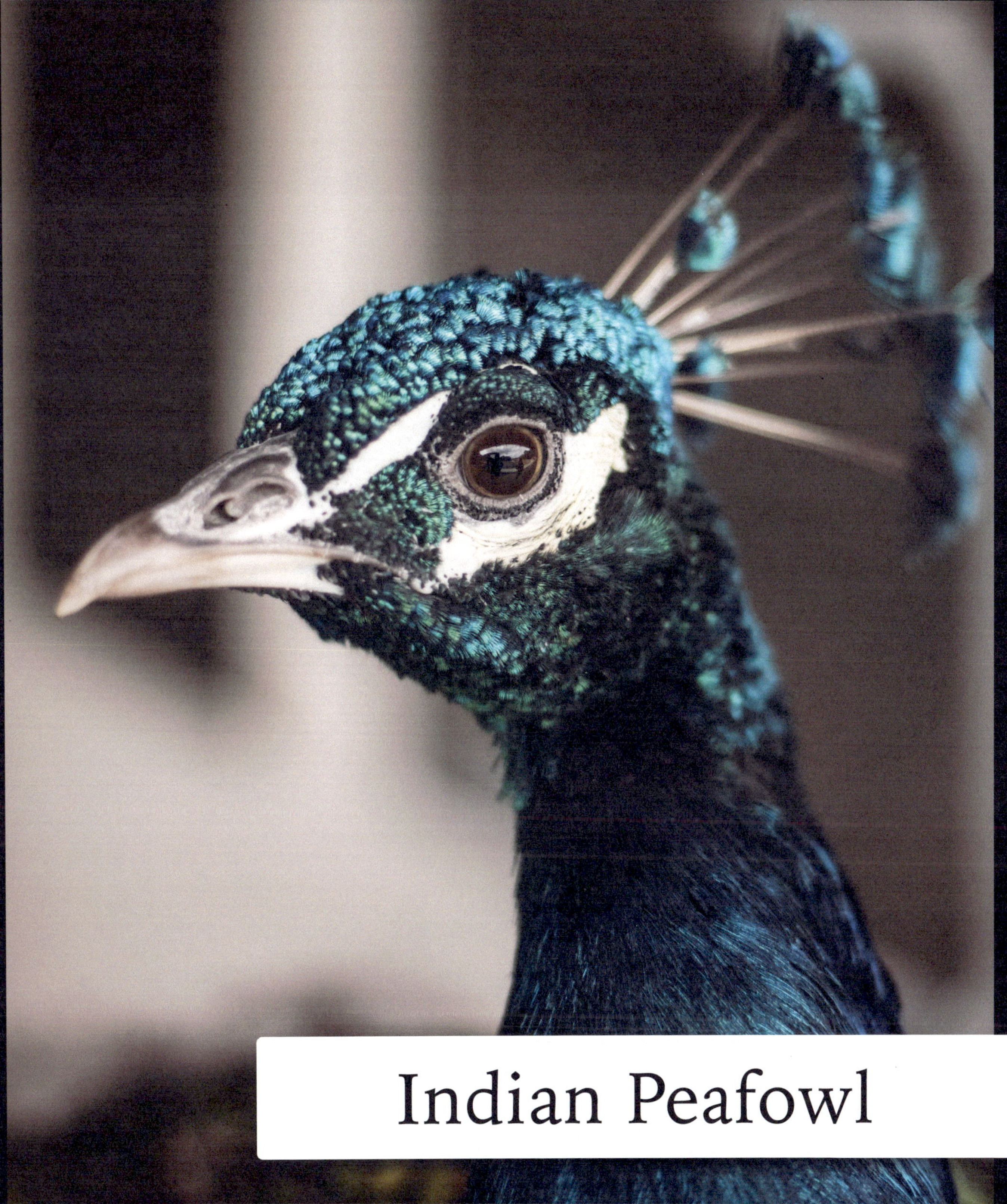

Indian Peafowl

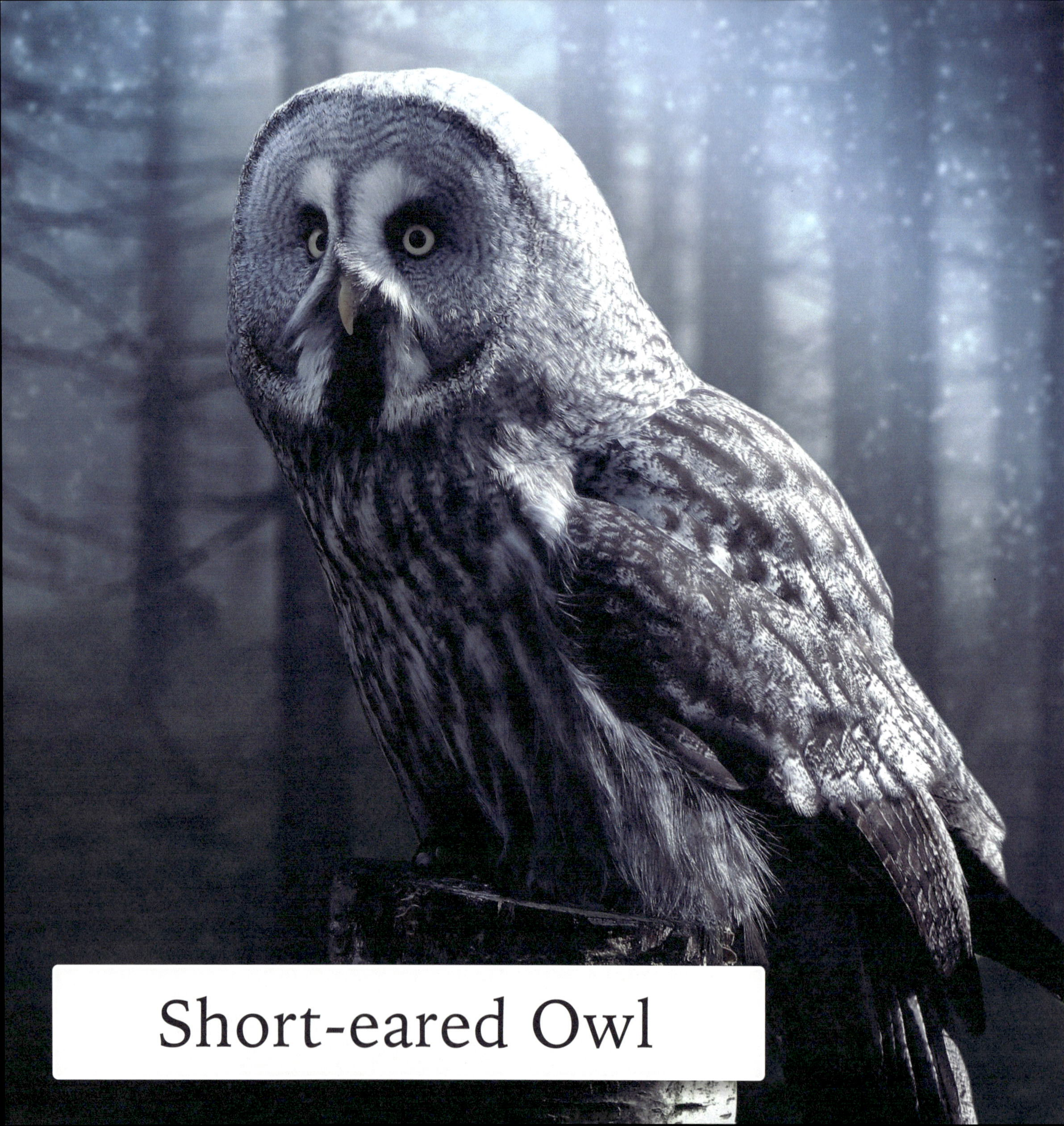

Short-eared Owl

Nilgiri Flycatcher

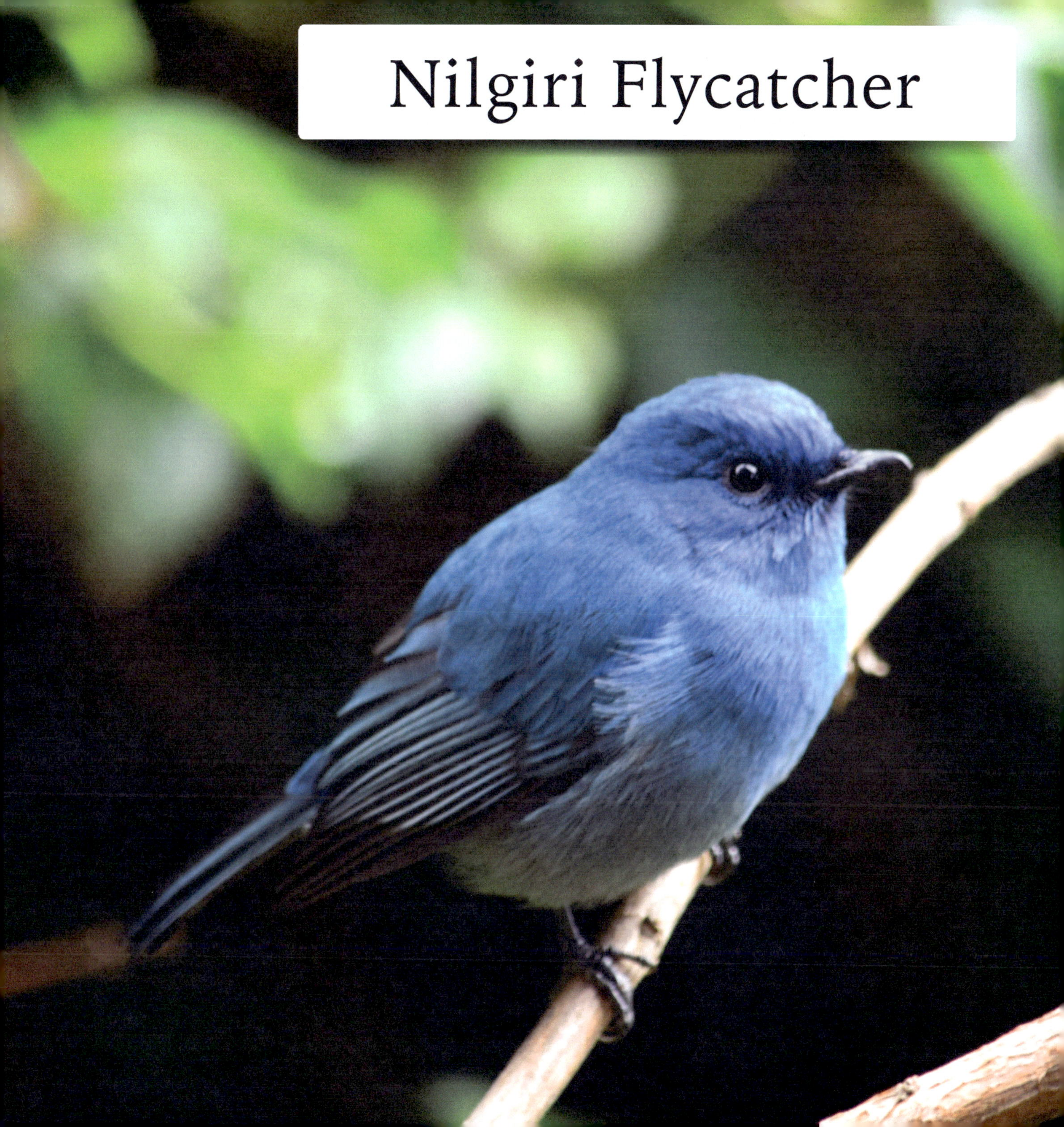

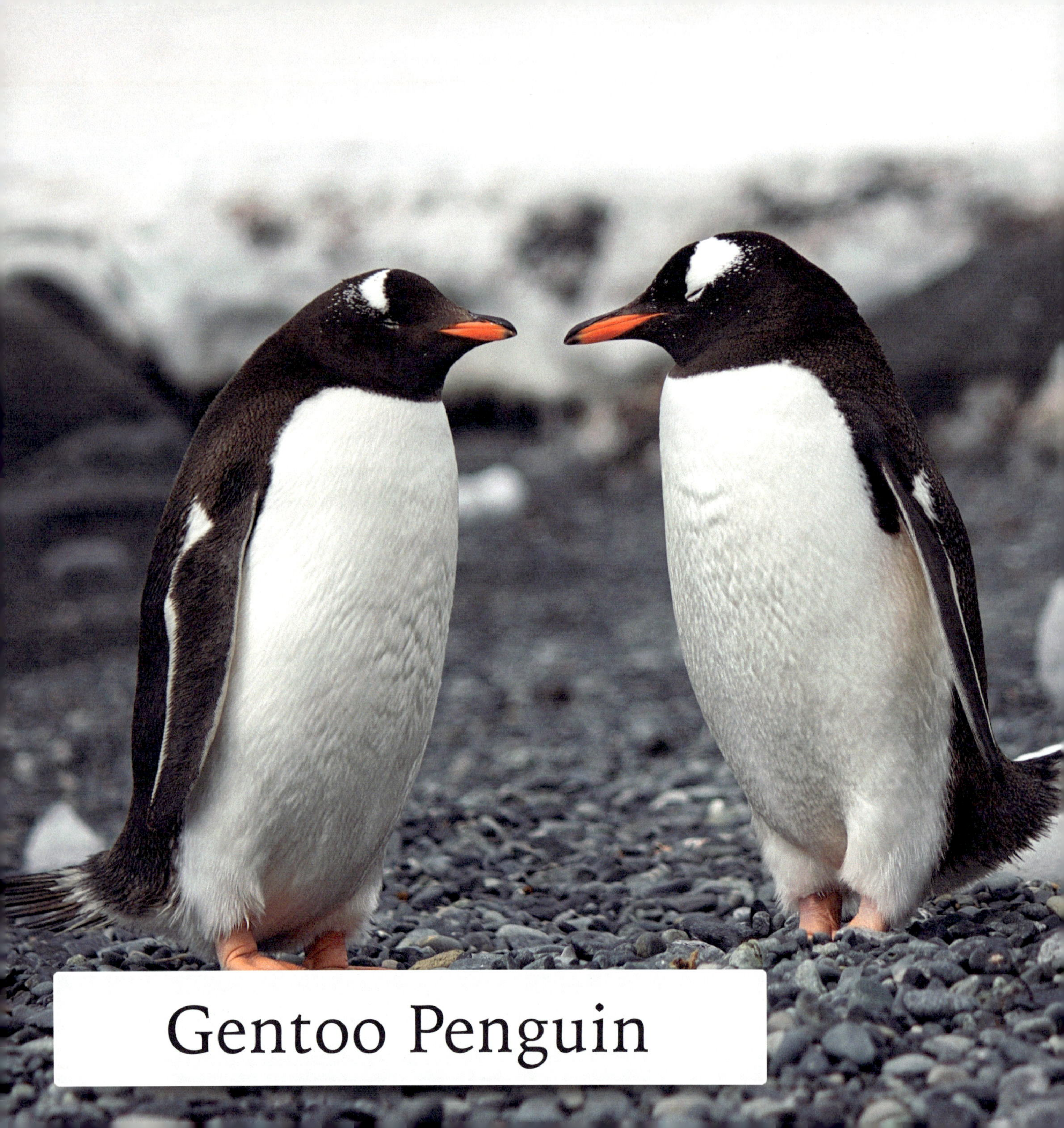

Gentoo Penguin

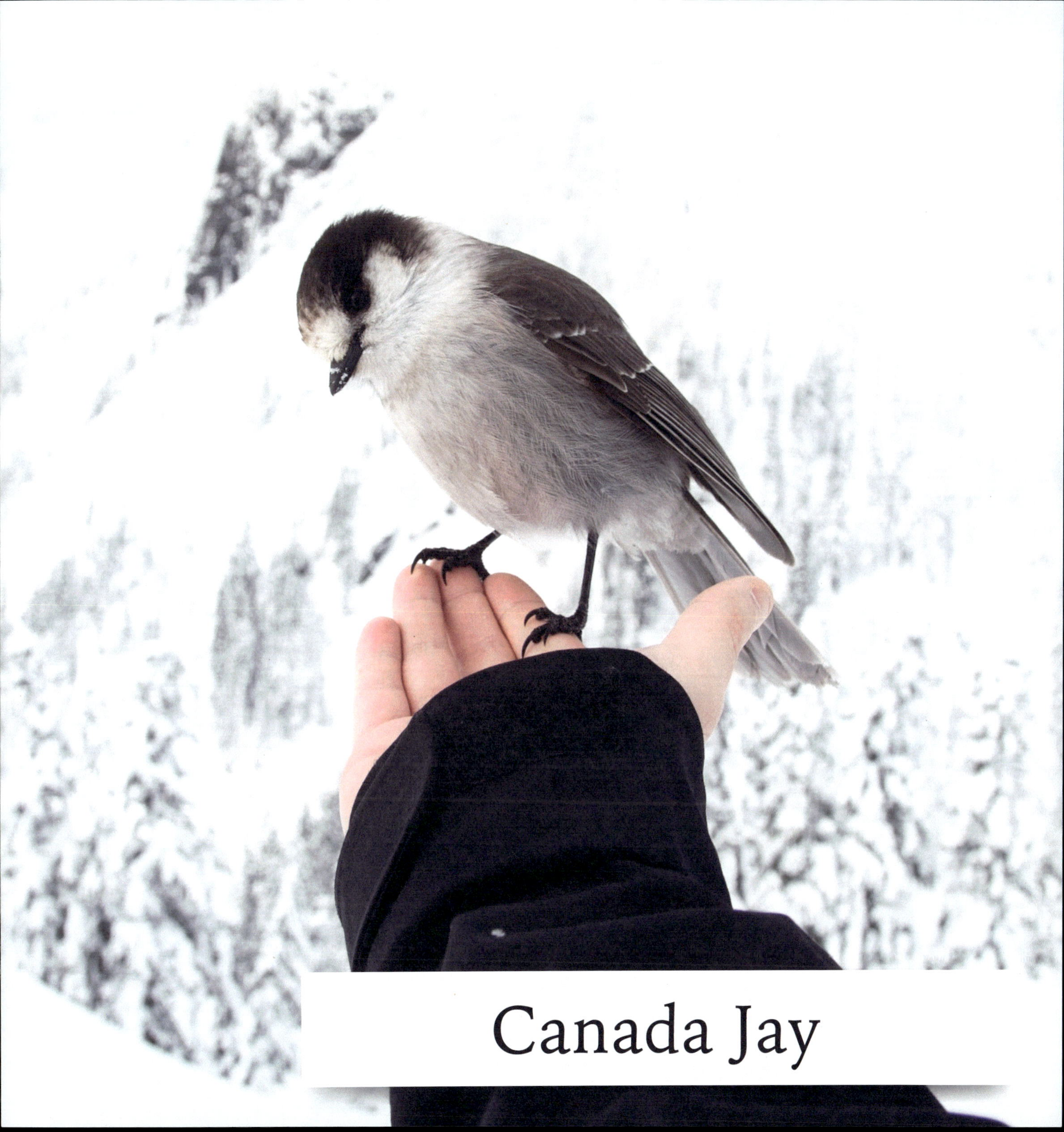

Canada Jay

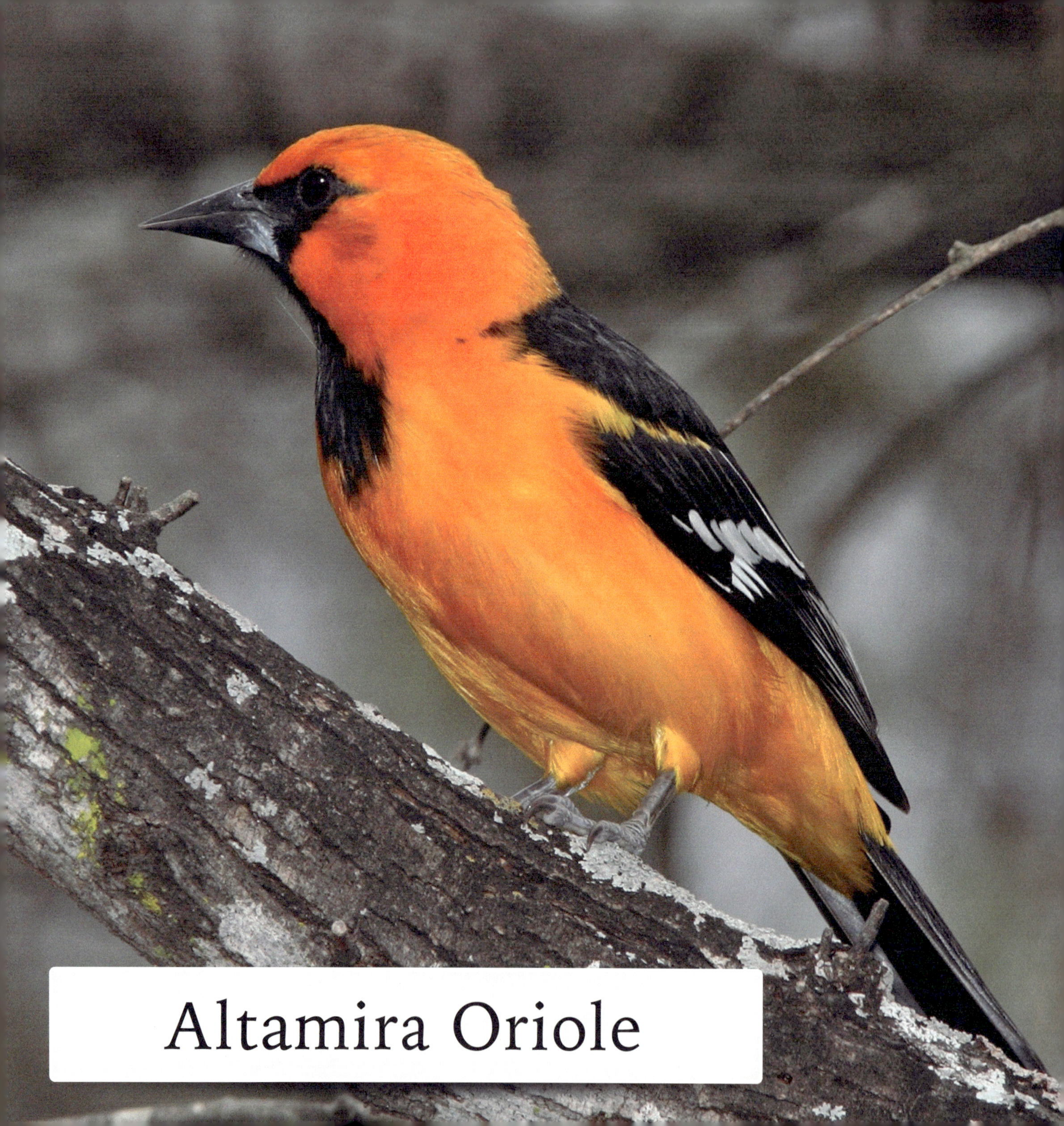

Altamira Oriole

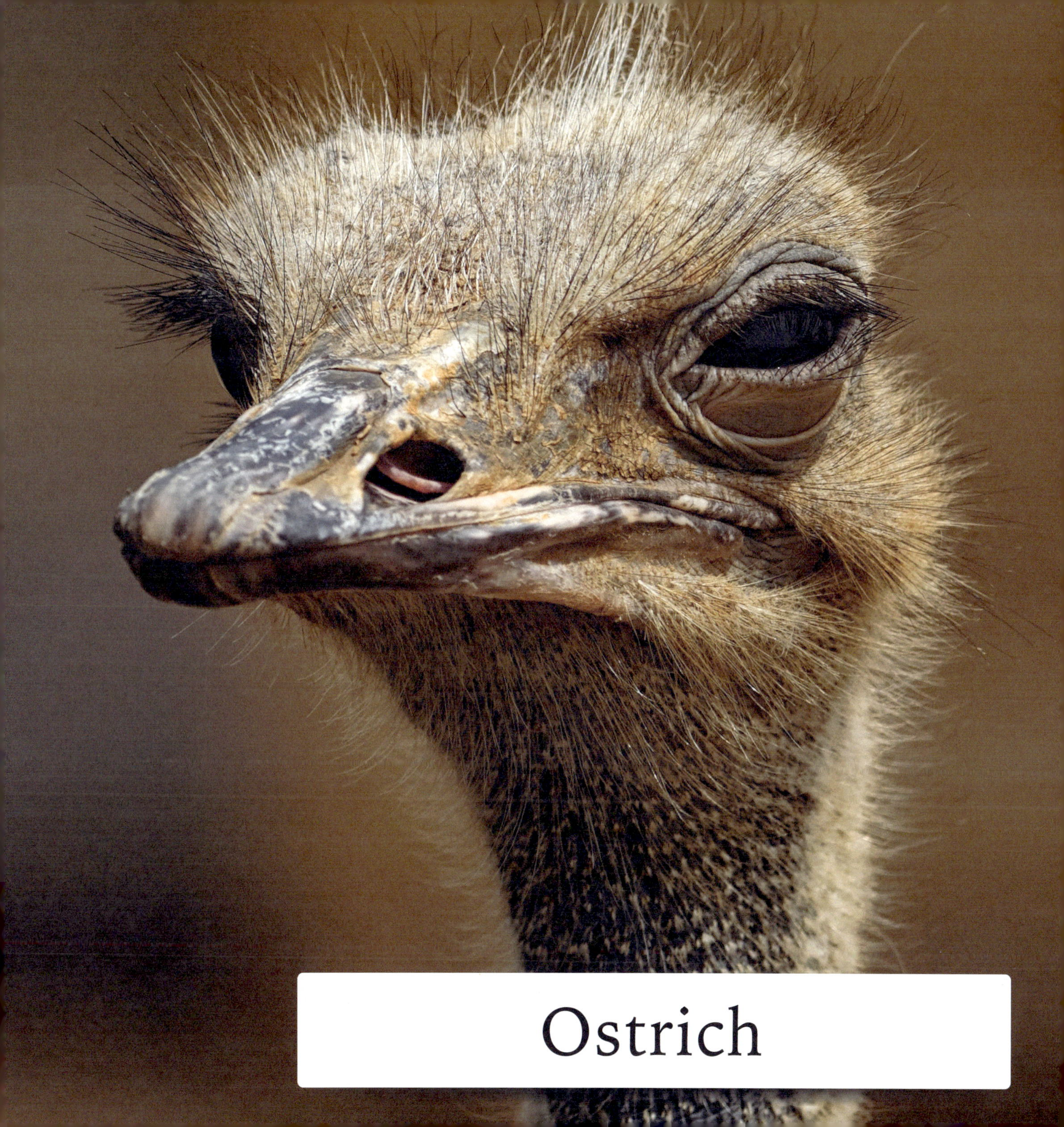

Ostrich

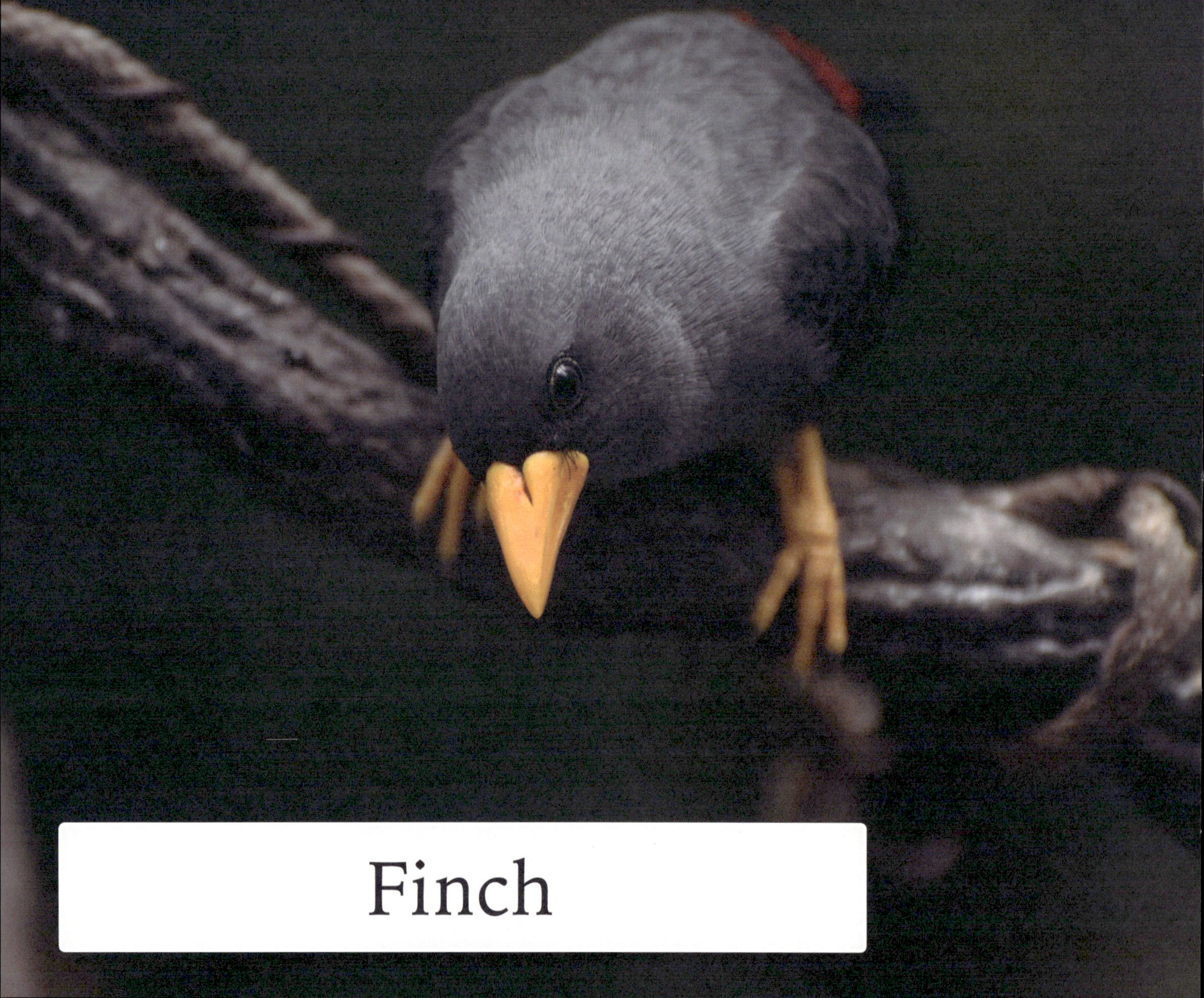

Finch

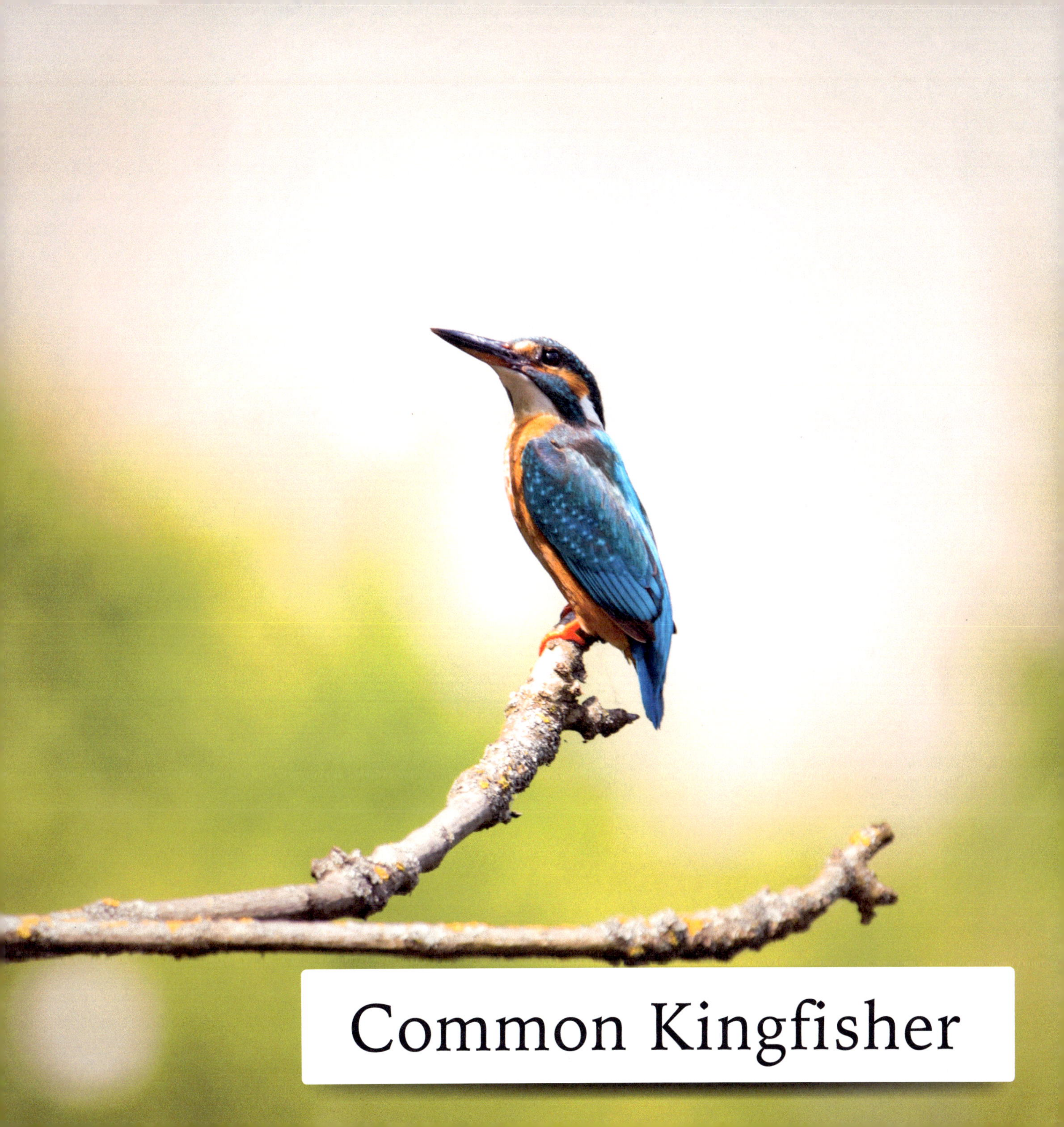

Common Kingfisher

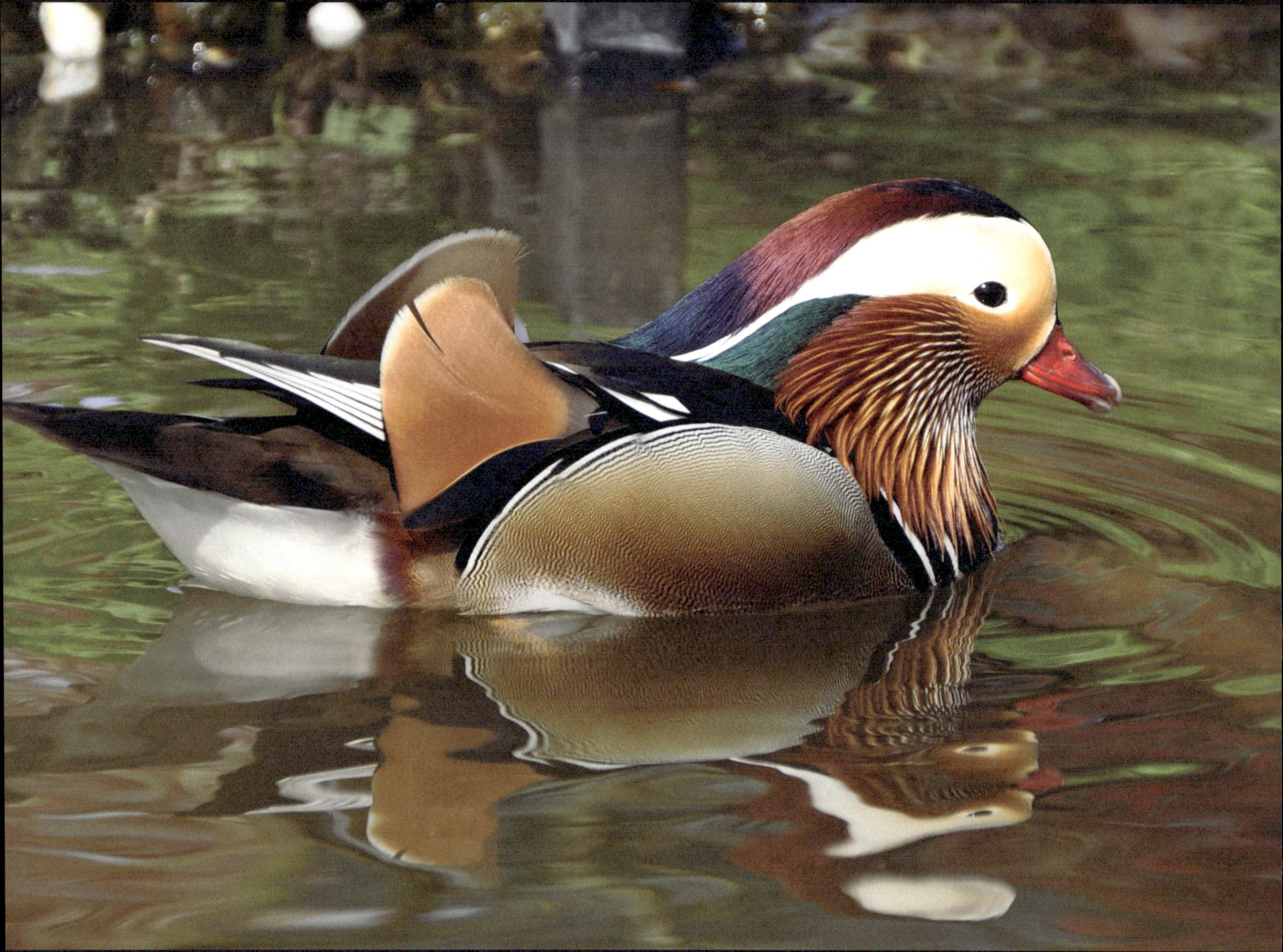

Mandarin Duck

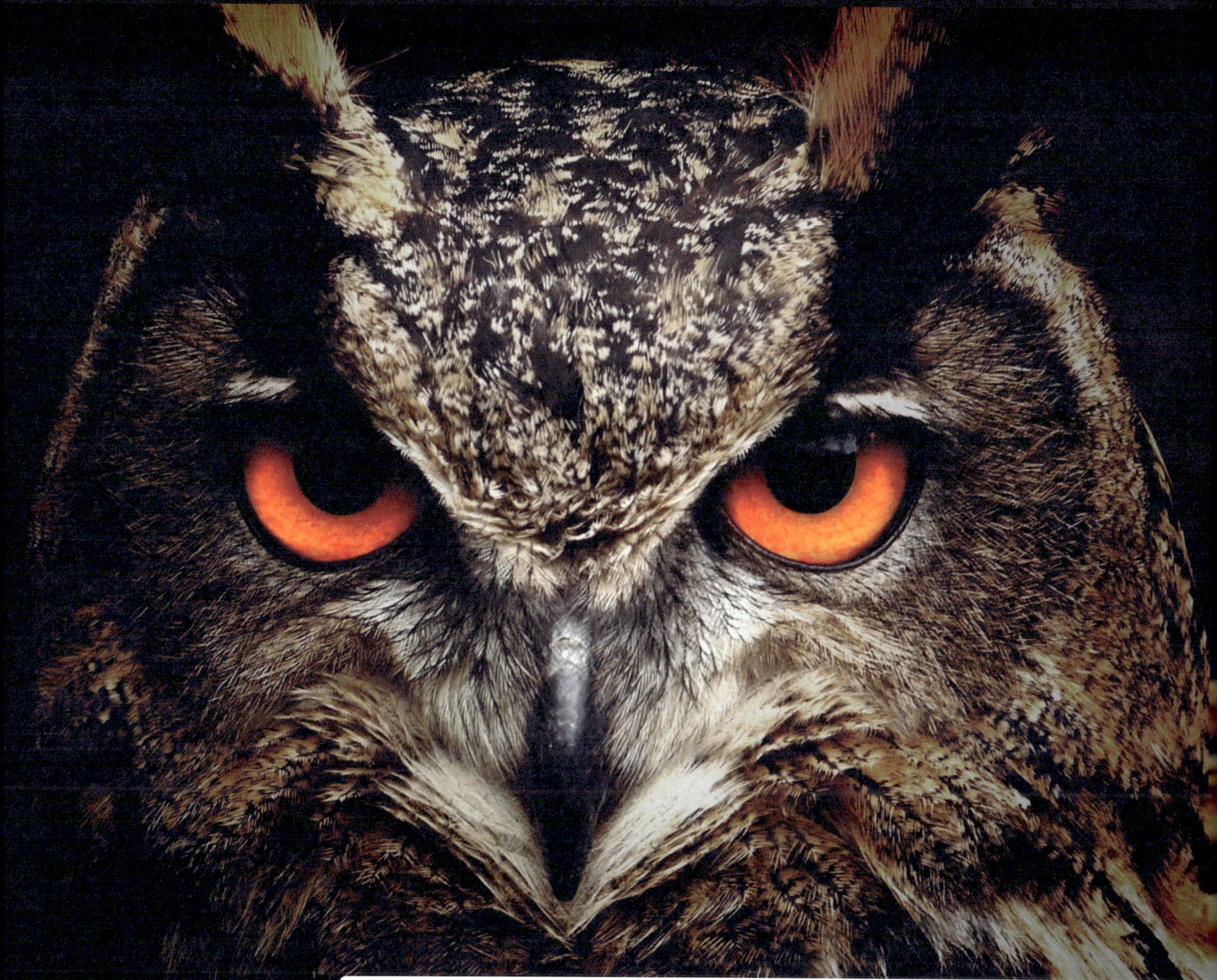

Eurasian Eagle-Owl

Rock Pigeon

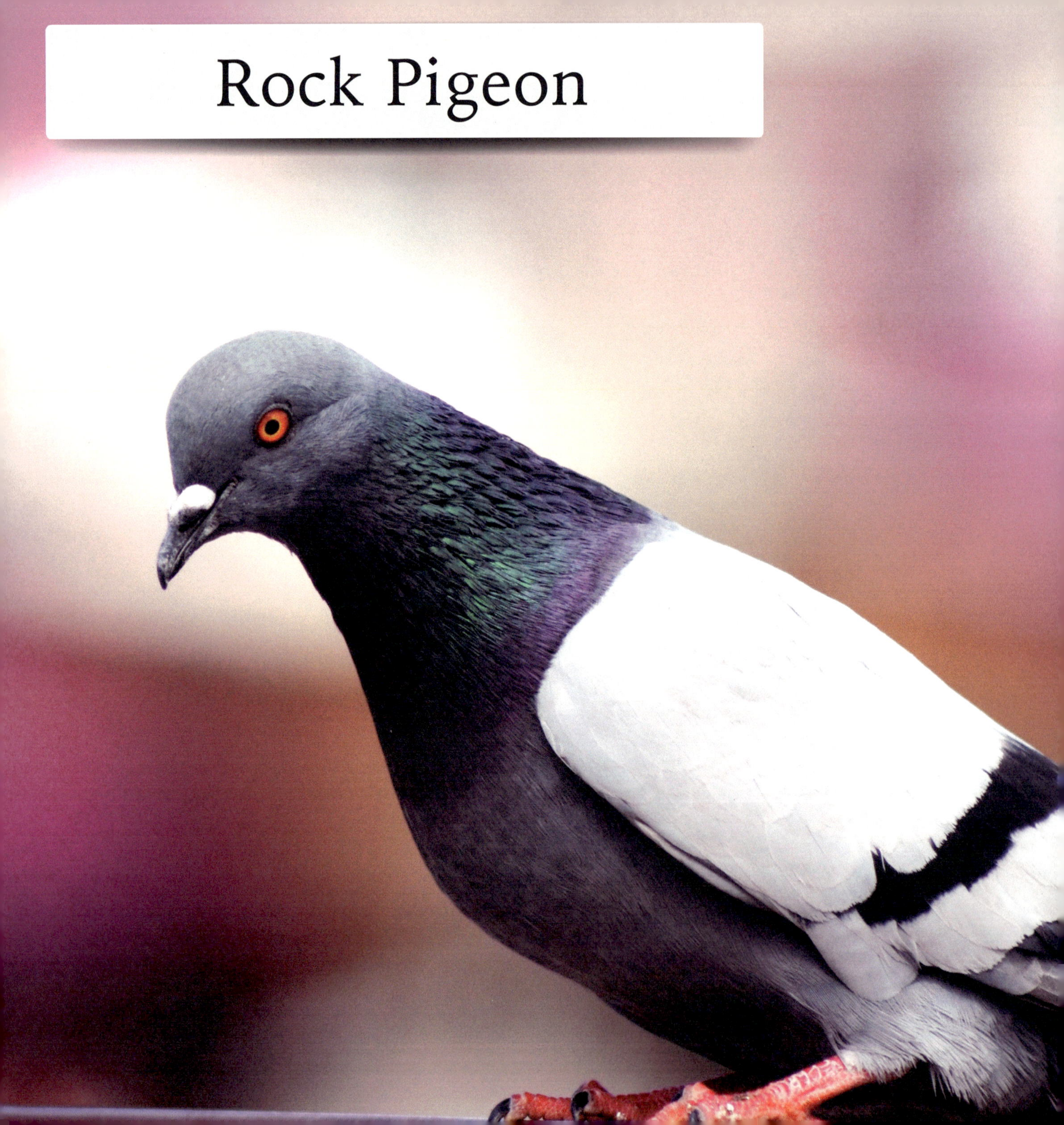

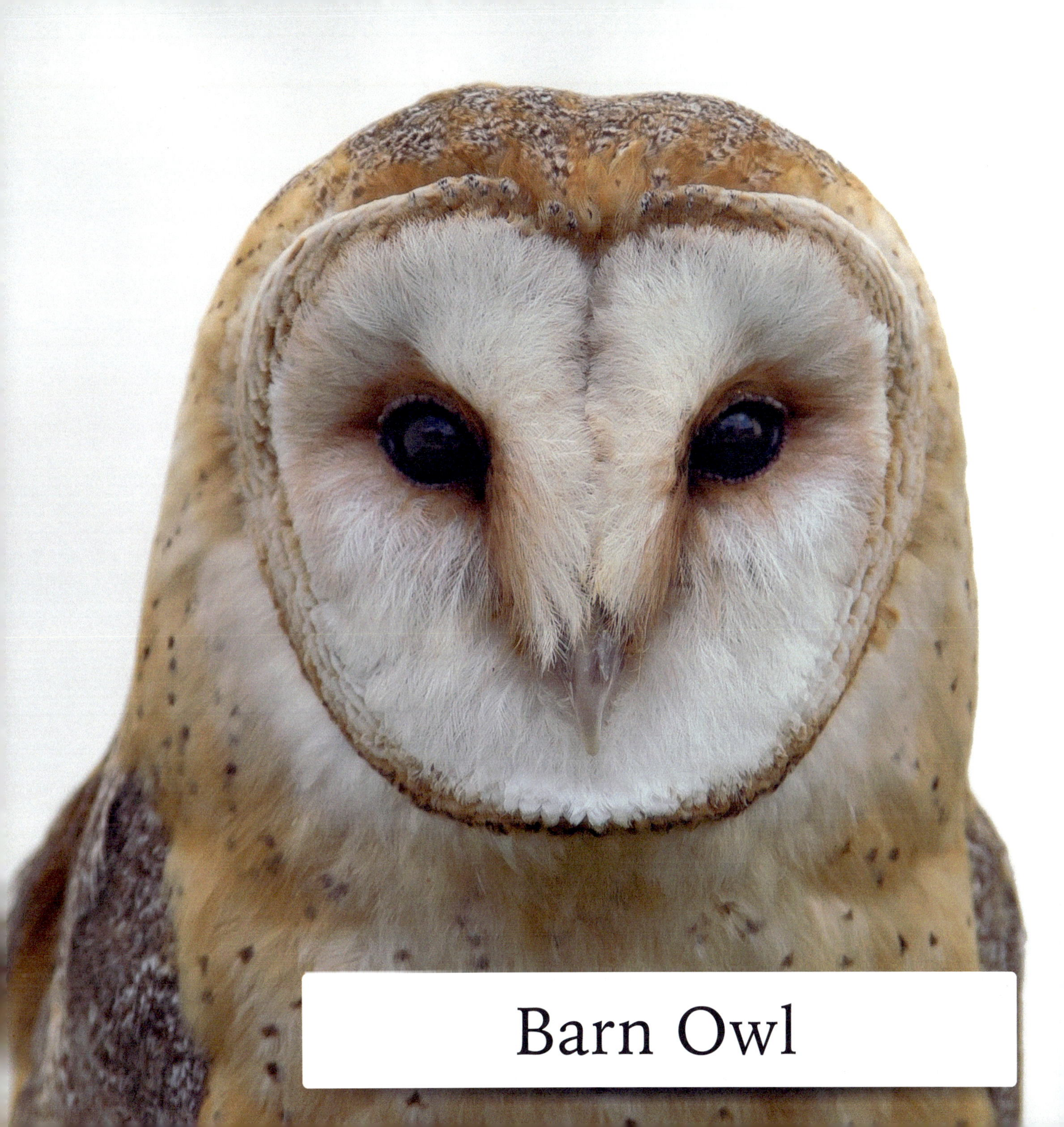

Barn Owl

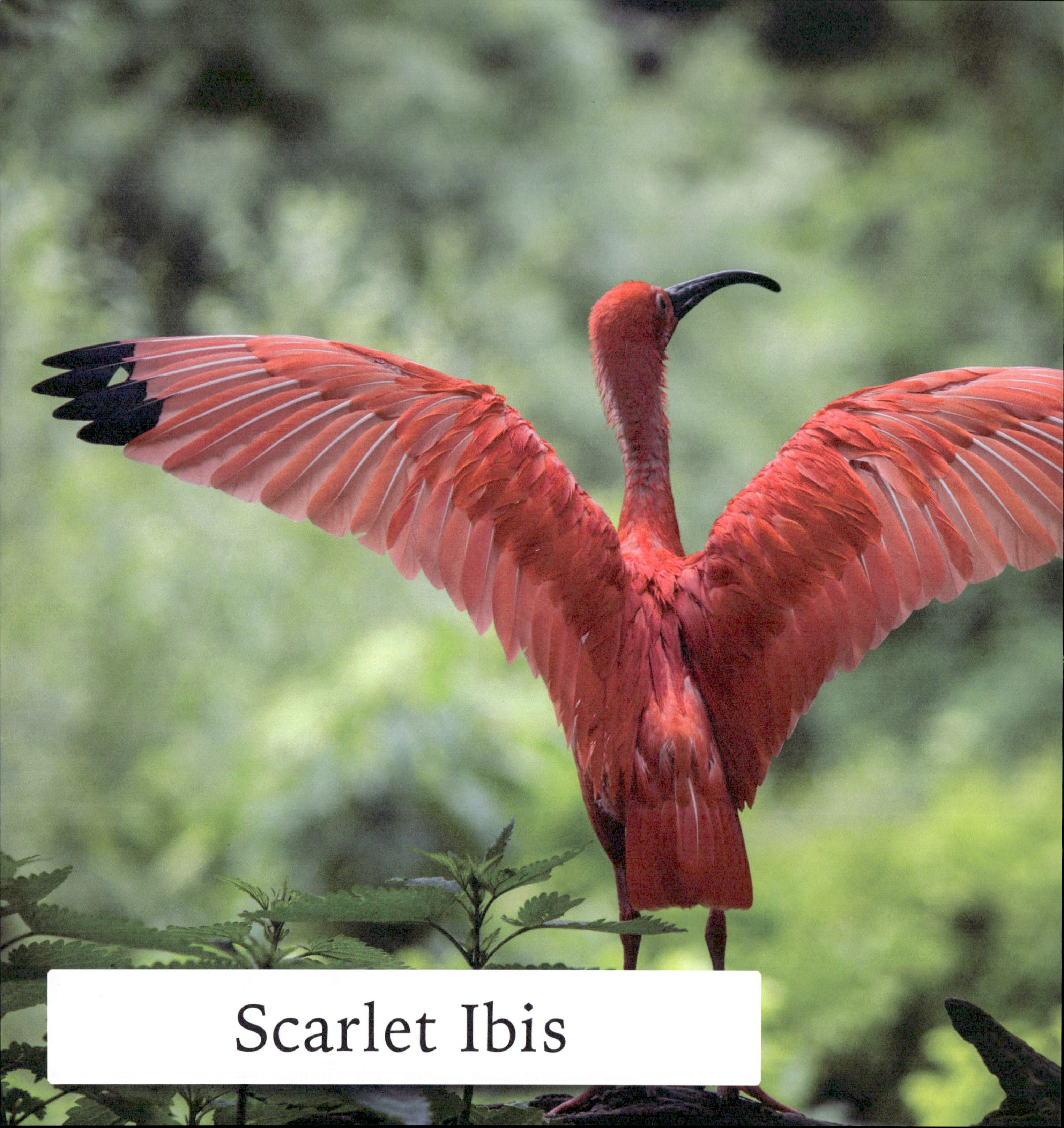

Scarlet Ibis

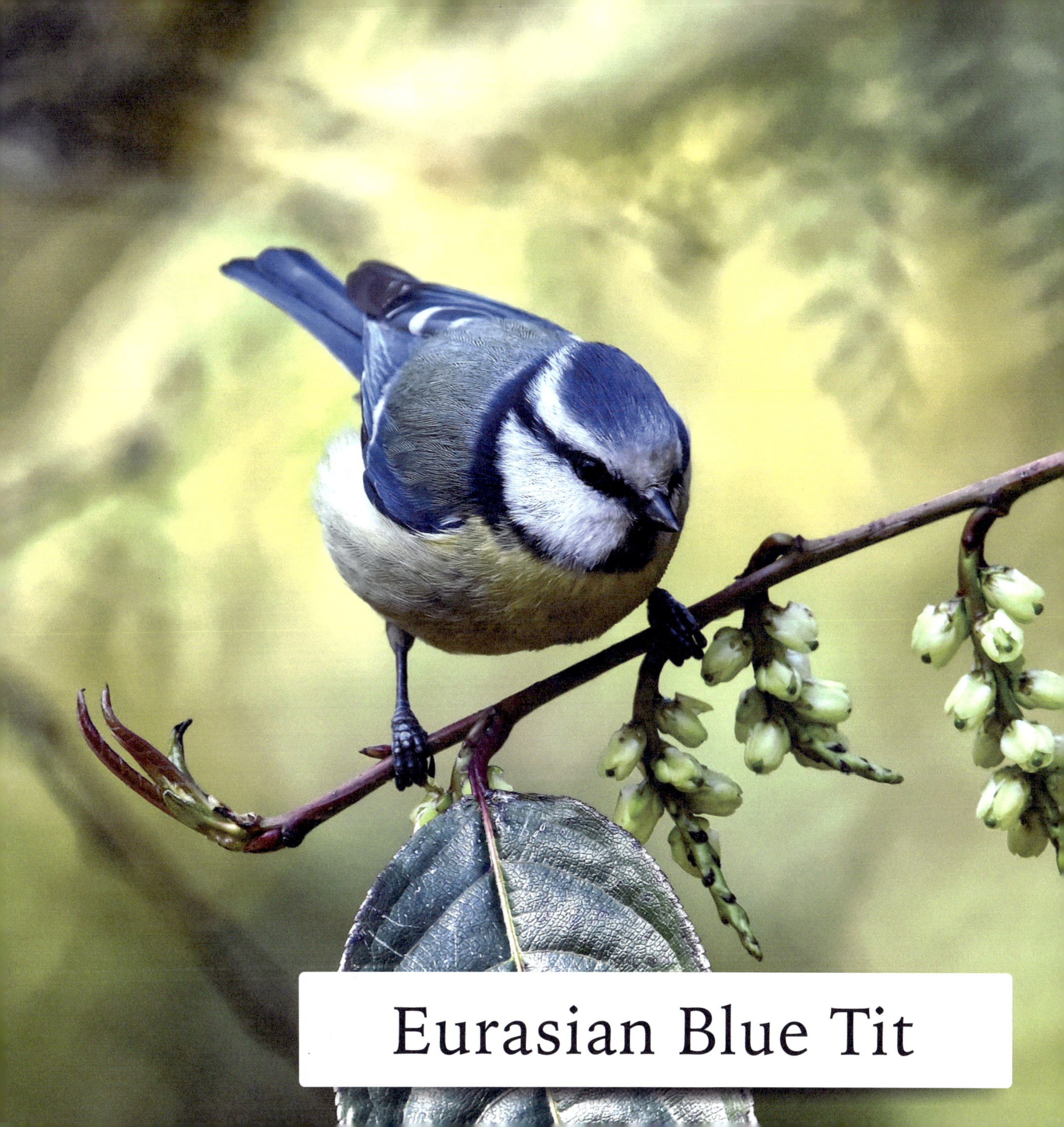

Eurasian Blue Tit

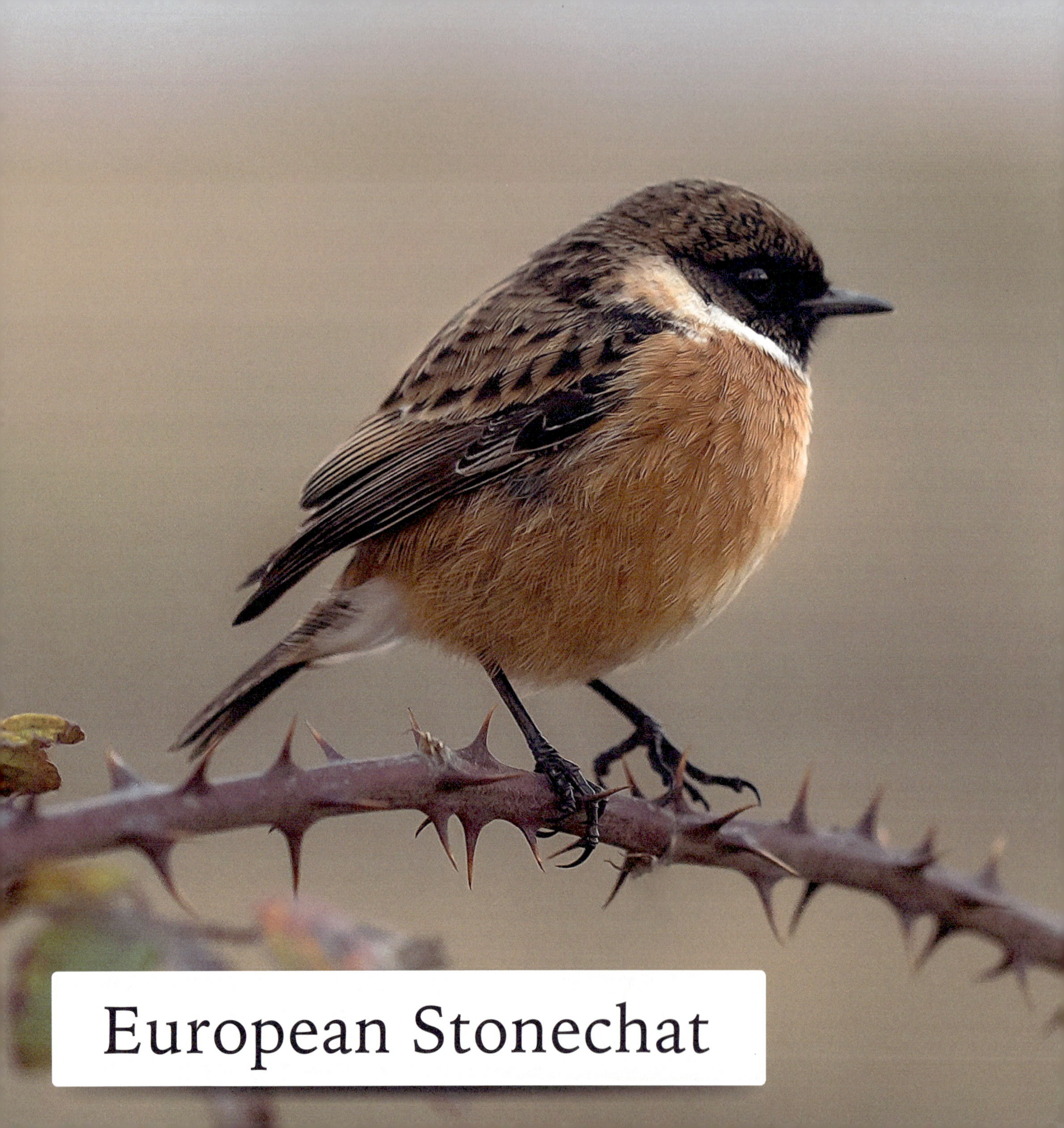

European Stonechat

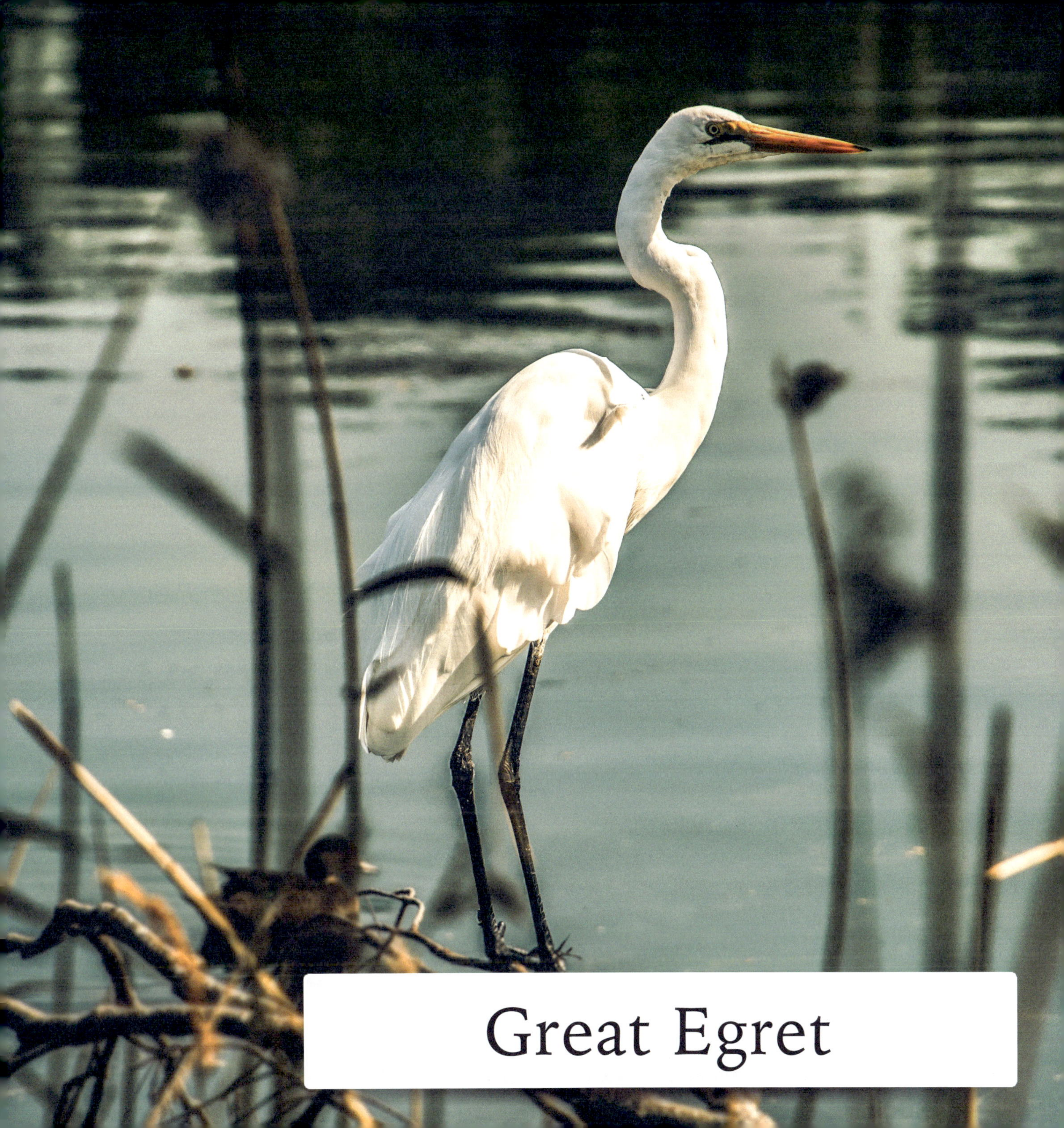

Great Egret

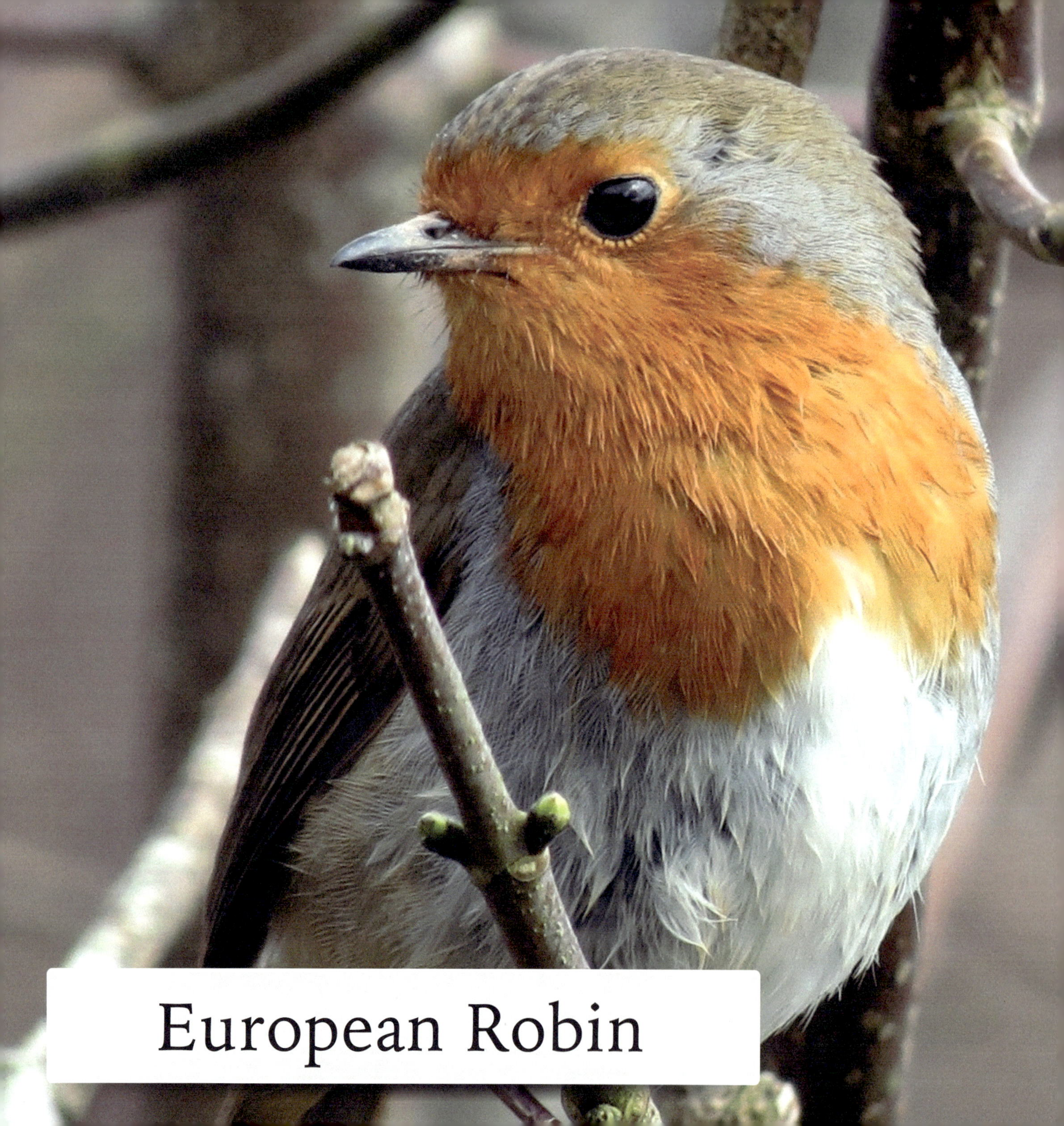

European Robin

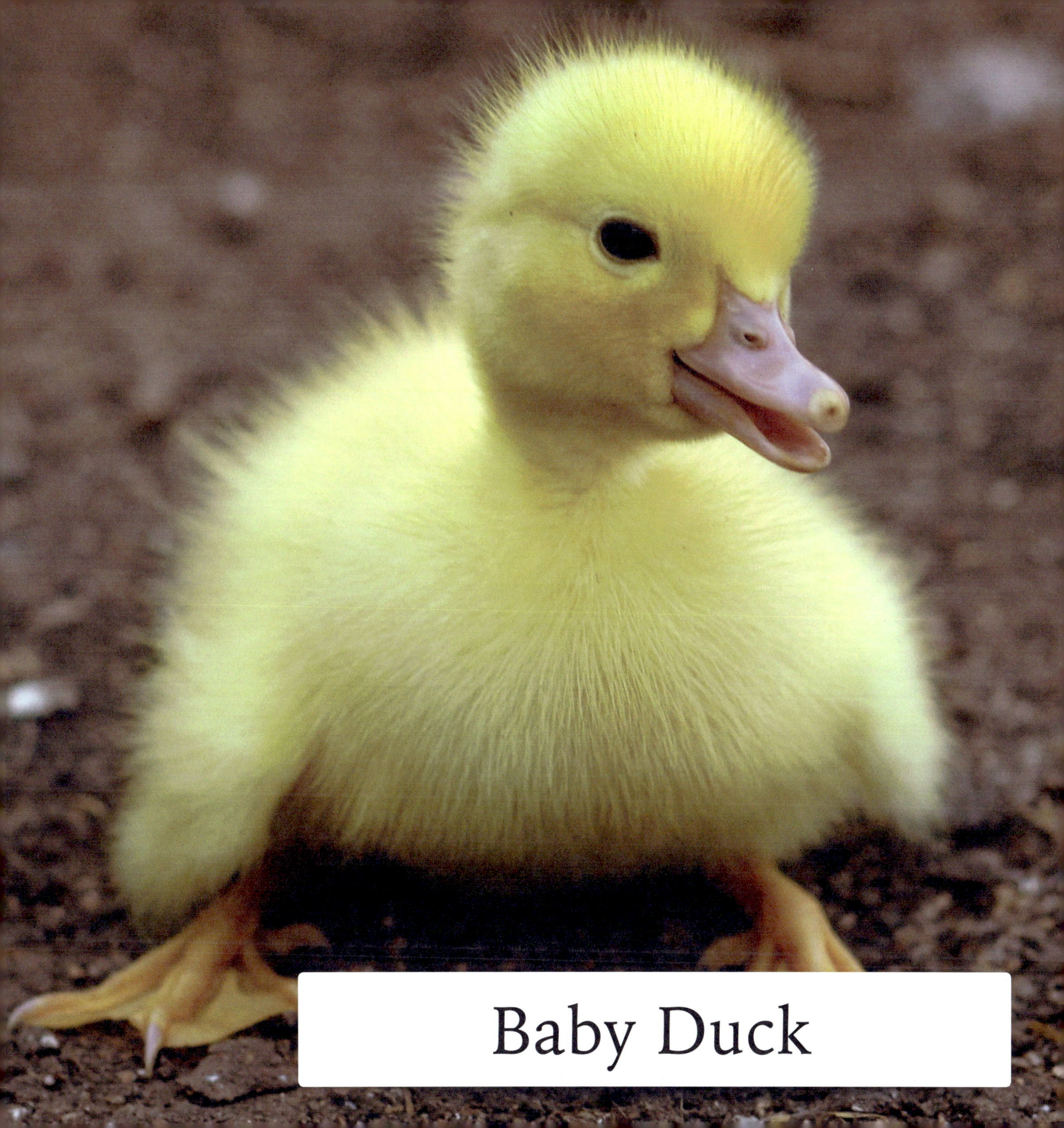

Baby Duck

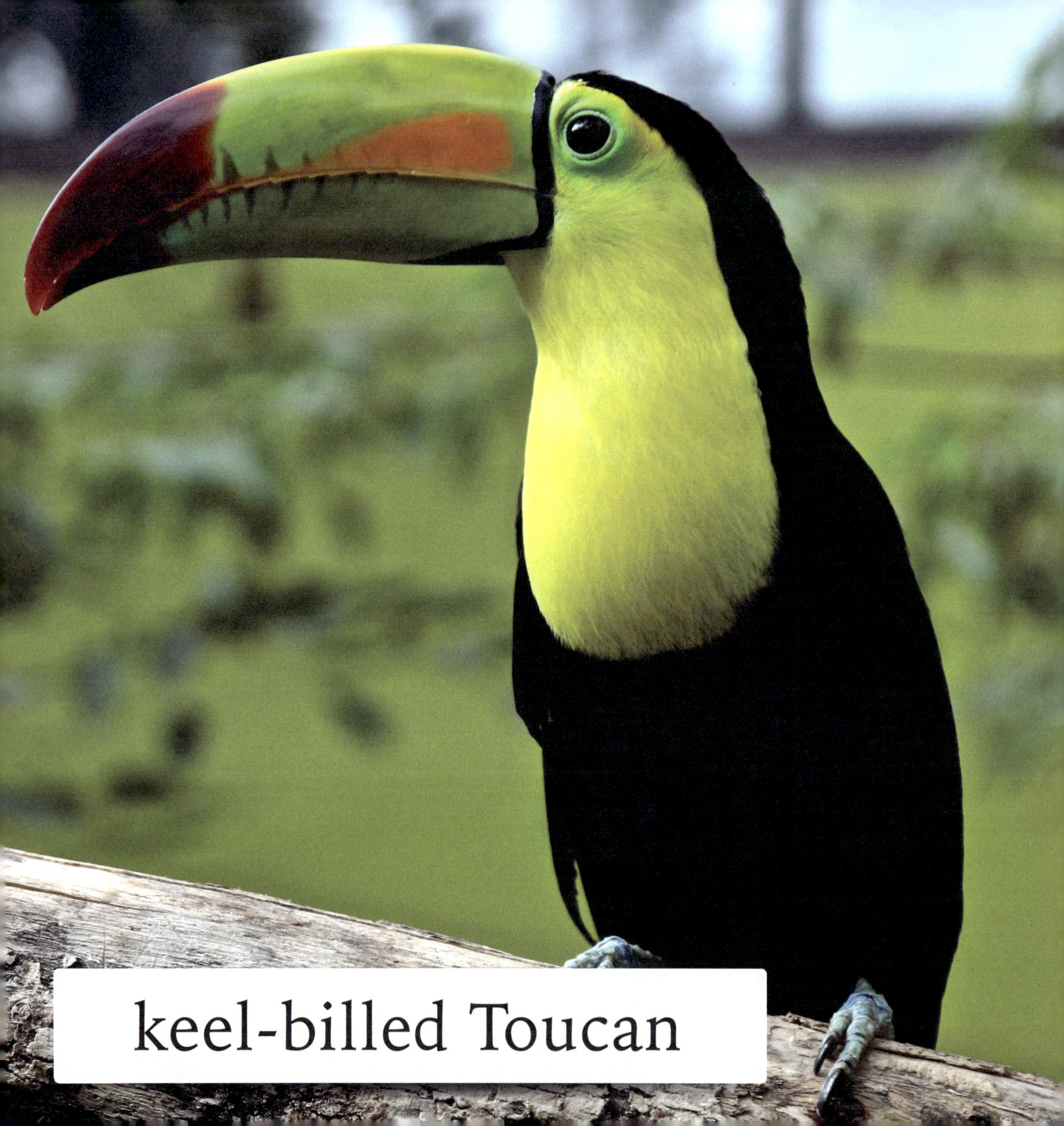

keel-billed Toucan

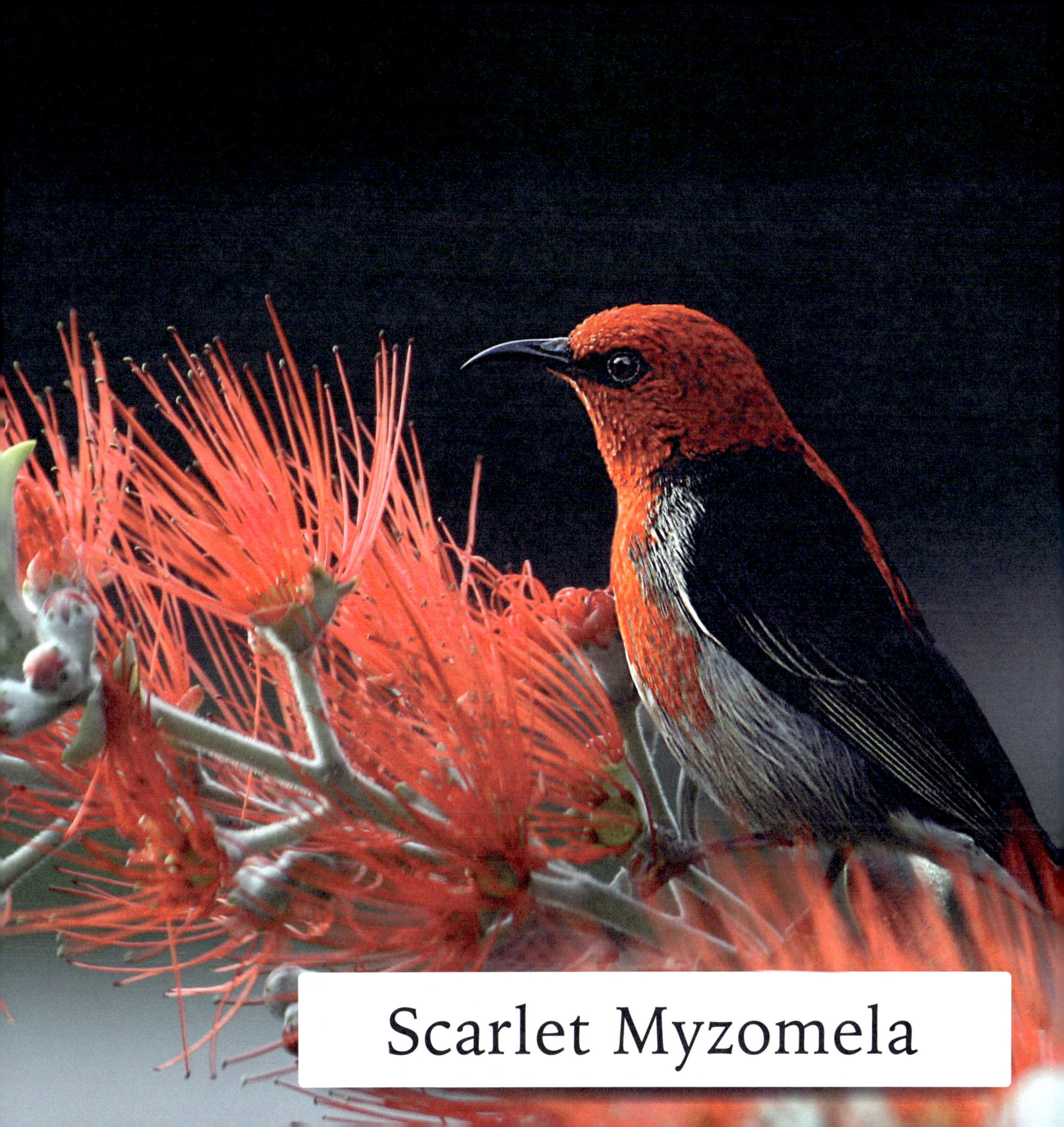

Scarlet Myzomela

Burrowing Owl

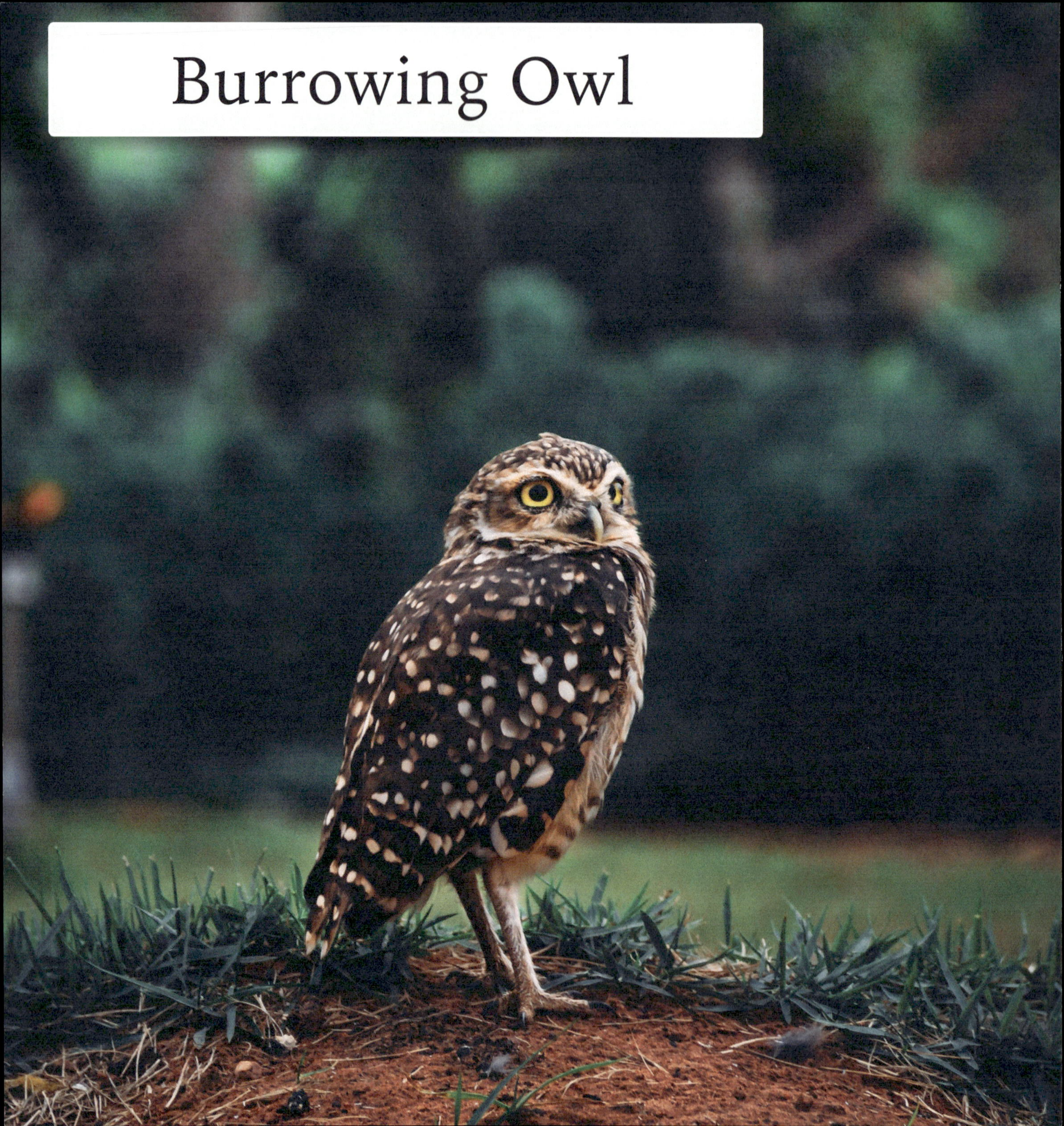

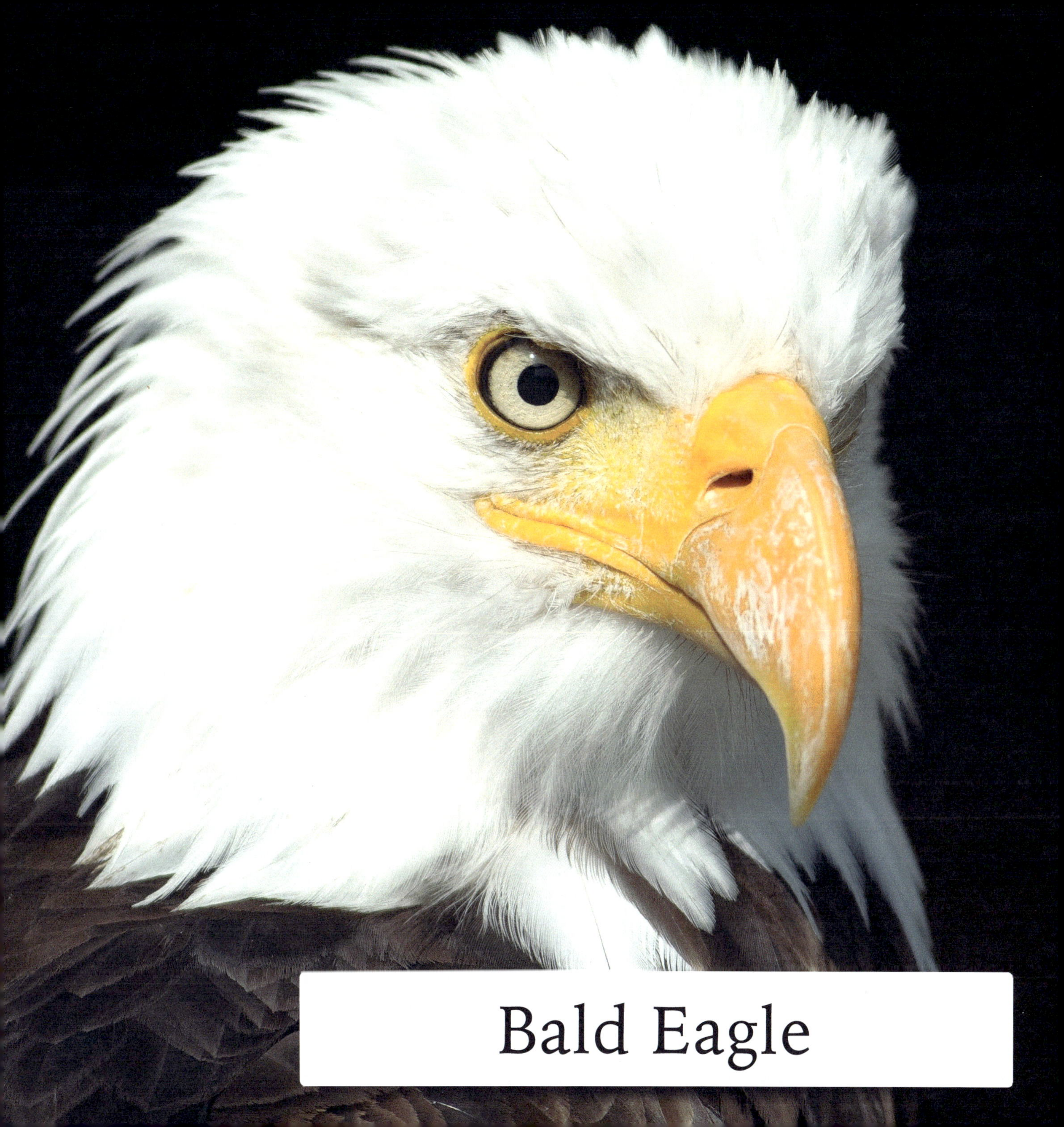

Bald Eagle

If you enjoyed this book please consider leaving a book review.

Your reviews really help us and others!

Mom And Son Prints

Thank You!

Please send us your feedback
or your book suggestions:
feedback@momandsonprints.com

MomAndSonPrints.com

Made in the USA
Las Vegas, NV
07 November 2026

57673303R00040